Massage for Therapists

MARGARET HOLLIS

MBE, MSc, MCSP, DipTP
Former Principal,
Bradford Hospitals School of Physiotherapy

BLACKWELL SCIENTIFIC PUBLICATIONS

OXFORD LONDON EDINBURGH

BOSTON PALO ALTO MELBOURNE

First published 1987
Reprinted 1988

Printed and bound by The Alden Press,
Osney Mead, Oxford

DISTRIBUTORS

USA
  Year Book Medical Publishers
  200 North LaSalle Street,
  Chicago, Illinois 60601
    (Orders: Tel. 312 726 9733)

Canada
  The C.V. Mosby Company
  5240 Finch Avenue East, Scarborough, Ontario
    (Orders: Tel. 416 298 1588)

Australia
  Blackwell Scientific Publications (Australia) Pty Ltd
  107 Barry Street, Carlton, Victoria 3053
    (Orders: Tel 03 347 0300)

British Library Cataloguing in Publication Data

Hollis, Margaret
  Massage for therapists,
  1. Massage
  I. Title
  615.8'22   RM721

ISBN 0-632-01757-0

Contents

Preface

When this book was first suggested to me I had considerable doubts whether I could describe massage in the written form in the same way as I had described it while demonstrating to my students for 40 years. I wanted the book to be readable and to be worked from so that the written word could become the action. Encouraged by many of my teaching colleagues of a wide age range I decided to go ahead provided that the book could be profusely illustrated. The photography involved many long sessions as we struggled to show an essentially moving skill at the most important and telling point of the movement. In this endeavour I have been fortunate to be able to work with Peter Harrison who brought his skill, endless patience and high standards to the task.

Equally patiently, Sheila Middlemiss modelled for me while Barbara Walker ticked endless lists and Janice Eccles again deciphered my writing to produce a coherent manuscript. I am grateful to each of them and also to the staff of the physiotherapy department at St Luke's Hospital, Bradford for the provision of facilities for the photography and for information about their recent experiences in treating the victims of the Bradford City Fire. If ever there needs to be justification for continuing to teach and learn massage the two ladies who allowed us to photograph some of their injuries being massaged would be the first to testify.

I now never undertake to write a book without the assurance that my trusted critic Barbara Turner will be available to read the manuscript; she has again fulfilled this role and I am greatly indebted to her. The staff of Blackwell Scientific Publications have continued to encourage me and I am grateful to them.

Finally I would like to express my thanks to the many hundreds of students of physiotherapy who, in learning massage in my practical classes and presenting me with their problems as they struggled to learn good techniques, taught me how to help them gain greater co-ordination so that they became practitioners of the art and skill of bringing a caring touch to help and comfort their patients. I hope the readers of this book will be able to achieve the same handling abilities.

Margaret Hollis

Note to the Reader

In this book the early chapters are intended for the student of massage who will I hope spend many hours practising on a model—hopefully a fellow student able to be aware of the 'feel' of the manipulations and thus able to comment constructively to the practitioner. The last chapter is about treatments for particular states or conditions. While these should be practised first on a model they will be used on patients or on sportsmen and sportswomen for specific effects. Thus in the early chapters I have referred to the recipient as the model and later on as the patient. Where techniques are practised on a model for use on a patient I have used both terms. I have hesitated to use the word 'client' which may be modern usage but can have unfortunate connotations in some circumstances! I have made the assumption that some knowledge of anatomy has already been achieved by my readers.

Chapter 1: Preparation for Massage

Massage is referred to by some people as an art, perhaps because its practice involves co-ordination of a high order and the use of great skill to achieve the integrated body movements which allow the application of the appropriate manipulations at the correct depth and speed to achieve maximum effect. To this end the potential practitioner must practise each manipulation with great awareness of their own contact with the subject, whether model or patient, so that any discomfort is immediately noticed and the cause detected. Uncomfortable massage is usually born of failure of co-ordinated performance by the practitioner. Minor adjustment of foot position and trunk posture will change the relationship of the practitioner to the support and the subject; and the totality of hand contact and the angle of contact will be altered by the posture of the trunk and arms. Finally, weight transference from the practitioner's feet to the subject will control depth. Rhythm must then be considered, as uneven movement of any one of the practitioner's body components will cause uneven contact, jerky movements of the whole line of work and angular patterns which will cause uneven compression or dragging by some part of the working hand.

Thus when starting to perform and practise massage check that you can:
- reach all parts,
- stand in walk or lunge standing to do so,
- change position from that shown in Fig. 1.1 to that shown in Fig. 1.2 without impedance or hesitation.

Self preparation

The practitioner should start preparation of himself or herself long before contact with the model/patient. Attention to personal appearance, hygiene and manicure are all important. As close contact will inevitably occur, the practitioner should wear protective clothing which is easily laundered and which allows freedom of movement while maintaining decency. Long hair must be restrained so that it cannot come into contact with the subject and, equally, necklaces or other jewellery which can dangle should be discarded as should a wristwatch. Rings should be removed as they can cause discomfort to the practitioner when performing some manipulations and to the model/patient during most manipulations. Thin wedding rings may be the exception to this rule—provided they do not cause discomfort to anyone. Well cared for hands which are smooth, with short, clean nails are essential.

Cleanliness is important so wash your hands before and after each treatment. Cultivate warm hands by always using warm water for washing and it also helps to keep your hands covered when outside in the cold.

The range of movements of all the joints of your forearm and hands should be full. If you have stiff hands, do a series of stretching exercises aimed at increasing your range of movement. The most important large range movements are:
- full abduction/extension of the thumb to give a wide grasp—an octave span

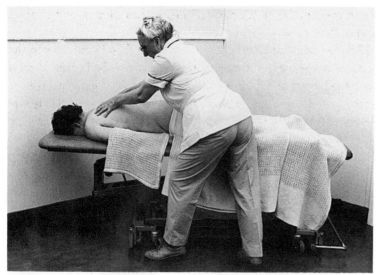

Fig. 1.1 Lunge standing reaching along the length of the body.

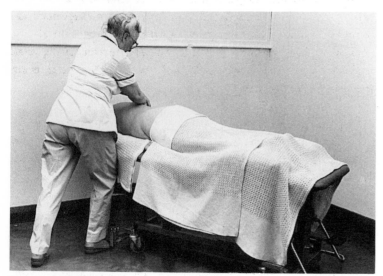

Fig. 1.2 Walk standing reaching across the body.

• full flexion and extension of the wrists or at least 80° of each movement

• full pronation and supination of the radio-ulnar joints.

Hand exercises

To obtain these ranges of movement the following exercises should be practised. Before each exercise check your shoulder relaxation:

1 Touch the finger tips of one hand with the finger tips of the other and press so that your thumbs and little fingers are separated widely.

2 Push the fist of one hand between two adjacent fingers of the other hand so that they are separated into wider abduction. Keep your fingers in the same plane. Repeat for each space (Fig. 1.3).

3 Place your hands together as in prayer and with your thumbs resting on your chest push your wrists downwards to extend them without separating the heels of your hands.

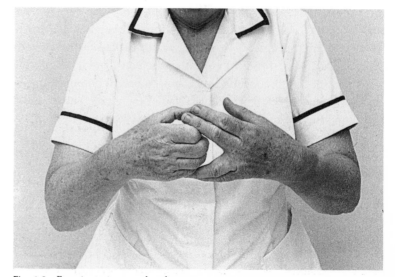

Fig. 1.3 Exercise to increase hand span.

4 Reverse your hands, placing the backs together and push your elbows downwards thus flexing your wrists.

5 Place your hands in the prayer position and, keeping them together turn them down and up. Try to touch your abdomen and chest alternately at each rotation. When you can hold the full extension with your hands just very slightly separated practise the rotation of your two hands, not touching, but simultaneously. Next move your two hands alternately so that they pass one another at mid-point (Fig. 1.4). Observe that the finger tips of each hand will now strike your abdomen at precisely the same point.

Relaxation

Relaxation of your hands is very important so that you always use your hands in full contact with your model/patient, and moulded to the shape of the body you are touching, with awareness of the tissues and of their state.

Relaxed hand contact is one in which the hand conforms to the contour of the part. The natural rest position of the human hand is with the fingers and thumb a little apart and very slightly flexed at each joint and it can easily be adjusted to allow contact with any size of body part. This is the contact which is used in many massage manipulations.

In addition you will need to be able to relax your whole arm to perform some manipulations. You should practise a method of relaxation yourself prior to learning massage. A good method is reciprocal relaxation as you will then become more aware of the position of all your joints and be capable of local relaxation of any body part as needed. Briefly, reciprocal relaxation involves working the opposite muscles to those you wish to relax, then stopping the action and appreciating the new, relaxed position of that body part.*

Co-ordinated and integrated movement of your body is essential for the comfortable and prolonged performance of massage manipulations without fatigue and physical stress on the practitioner.

You should stand in walk standing and practise transferring your weight forwards and backwards while maintaining your arms stretched away from you:
- across the couch as in Fig. 1.2;
- along the couch as in Fig. 1.1.

These movements, along the length of the model/patient and across the model/patient, are key movements in massage. The former allows you to practise long, reaching actions with variable weight from your hands on to the length of the body structures; the latter allows you to practise short, reaching actions with variable weight from your hands across the length of the body structures.

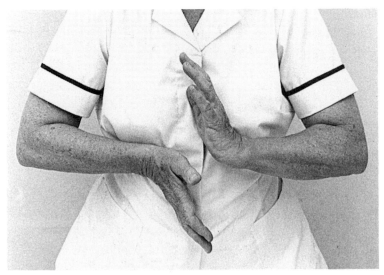

Fig. 1.4 The ultimate ability is to maintain wrist extension with a relaxed hand and perform full range pronation and supination with alternate hands.

*See Hollis M. (1981) *Practical Exercise Therapy*, 2nd edn, pp. 33–4. Blackwell Scientific Publications, Oxford.

The environment

The treatment area should be well heated and well ventilated but not draughty. The padded treatment couch may be covered with fresh linen.

Linen you may need

- An underblanket and a covering cotton sheet
- Large and small washable blankets and/or sheets
- Standard size pillows and pillow covers
- Small or half size pillows and pillow covers

Treatment couch

An adjustable height couch is most useful, of the type that has an elevating mechanism at each end and a removable section to accomodate the nose when the model/patient is in prone lying. The couch should be covered with an underblanket if it is made of 'cold' material, with a cotton sheet on top. You may find it more manageable to anchor these covers with a series of flat straps, checking that the fastenings are under the couch and not in contact with the model/patient.

Contact materials

Powder

- Talcum powder is the commonest contact medium. It should be non-perfumed if possible, or a baby powder may be selected.
- Corn Starch BP, which is sterilizable, is a heavy powder which absorbs sweat very readily and should be used in the presence of profound sweating by either the model/patient or the practitioner.

Oils

- Pure lanolin—which has a 'drag' effect on skin due to its thick and heavy texture is used to obtain a slight pull on the skin. Lanolin cream which is a water based cream is used when less 'drag' is required.
- Liquid oils—the most commonly used liquid oil is probably Ol.arachis (nut oil) but olive oil or liquid paraffin may also be used to provide a 'gliding' effect and to lubricate the skin. The disadvantage of such oils is that they become rancid and, if left in contact with the skin can smell offensive.

Water-based lubricants

The water-based lubricant most commonly used is ung. eucerin. This light cream is used to give moderate lubrication and, as it absorbs rapidly, is mainly of value as an introduction to deeper work.

The thinner oils used in massage tend to reduce the depth at which the practitioner can work as the hands glide on the lubricated skin and slide away from the part being treated, instead of working with depth. Thicker oils do not cause this problem. Note also that the smaller the manipulations you perform when using oils, the more likely you are to obtain greater depth.

Soap and water

Soap and hot water, with or without the addition of oil is used for scaly skins which may be caused by prolonged immobilization in a plaster cast or by use of some medications which promote and increase skin healing and at the same time cause the skin to become dry and scaly.

Preparation of the patient/model

Ask the patient/model to undress so that the part to be treated is adequately uncovered. Remember that some manipulations, to be effective, must extend to the lymph glands lying in proximal spaces. Thus:

For treatment of the upper limb, unclothe from the neck to finger tips and especially remove all straps.

For treatment of the lower limb, unclothe from the groin to the toe—*remove* trousers, do not pull them up.

For treatment of the back, unclothe from the head to the buttocks. Pants/briefs can remain on, but must be pulled down to leave the area above the gluteal cleft exposed.

For treatment of the neck, unclothe from the head to the level of the lowest point of origin of trapezius, i.e. 12th thoracic vertebra.

For treatment of the face, unclothe from the hairline to just below the clavicle.

Ensure the patient/model is kept warm by the use of blankets, e.g. if he or she is sitting, wrap him or her in a blanket leaving the arm part to be treated free (Fig. 2.3). If the patient/model is to lie down cover him or her immediately, having first placed pillows in position as needed. The patient in lying may need:
- one or two head pillows
- a pillow under the knees (Fig. 2.16).

The patient in prone lying may need:
- two head pillows crossing one another to create an inverted and open triangle so that his or her nose rests below the crossing
- a pillow under the abdomen to raise and thus flatten the lumbar spine (Fig. 6.1)
- a pillow under the ankles to flex the knees slightly.

More pillows will be needed for special positions and these are dealt with in the treatments section.

If you use one large blanket initially ensure that smaller blankets are on hand so that you can split the covers to keep the patient/model covered and warm.

Small sheets are very useful for placing in direct contact with the patient/model and to protect the blankets. Sheets are more easily washed and less likely to retain any powder you may use.

Palpation and developing sensory awareness*

Palpation is a skill that is acquired by practice. It requires that your hands should be relaxed, in firm comfortable contact, and aware of what is under them. The term 'thinking hands' implies that your mind is envisaging the structures that your hands are feeling and is alert both to identify the structure and become aware of variations from normal of the state of the structure.

To learn how to palpate, practice the following procedures. Place your whole hand on a series of varying size, rounded structures in turn, starting with large ones that require an almost flat hand, for example:
- a cushion or part-filled hot water bottle
- a smaller bottle or rolling pin
- a broomstick handle.

Increase your pressure on the object to grasp firmly with your whole hand, modifying your hand posture so that every part of the palmar surface is in contact simultaneously. Then release your pressure very slowly until you are only just grasping—think hard about the quality of this pressure. Next, release your pressure so that the object could start to slip. Think about and appreciate this pressure, as such pressure is likely to tickle the patient.

Following this, enlist the help of a colleague and repeat the procedure, applying in turn very firm, firm and very light contact on the

*From Hollis, M. & Yung, P. (1985) *Patient Examination and Assessment for Therapists*, pp. 12–15.

putting only your finger tips on again. To do so will cause you either to poke and hurt or to tickle by touching again too lightly. Remember that too hard a pressure will feel like a drill digging in (Fig 1.5) and too light a pressure will feel like a butterfly coming to rest (Fig 1.6). In neither case will you feel or find anything.

Now slide your fingers towards the structure to be palpated and in doing so ensure that your pressure is such that you neither drag the

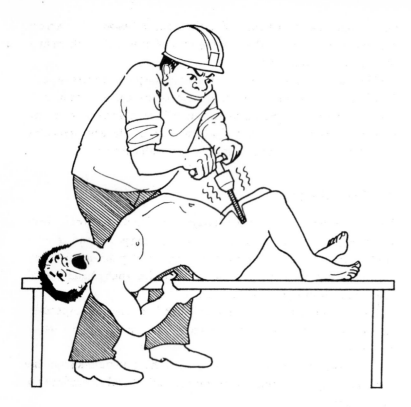

Fig. 1.5 Do not palpate at the depth of a drill.

back, the thigh, the calf, the arm, the forearm and the foot. Appreciate what pressure/contact you need to be able to touch and not hurt, and to touch and not tickle.

Again use a colleague and decide to palpate for specific anatomical features. Place more of your hand than you need in contact with the area to be examined, lift your palm a little to reduce the contact, so that only the finger pads are touching firmly enough. Your fingers should be straight so that your nails are unlikely to be in contact. Do not lose contact, but, if you do, refrain from re-establishing it by

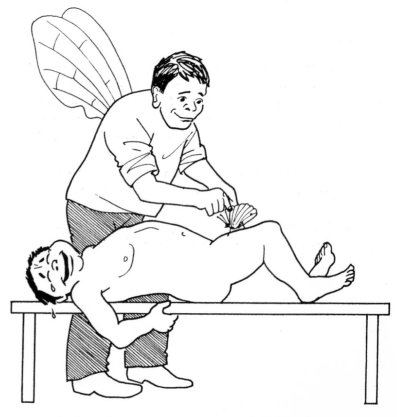

Fig. 1.6 Nor feel like a butterfly.

skin nor skid over it. Mentally count off the anatomical landmarks and apply the check tests that you have learned for identifying that structure, for example:

1 arteries can be felt to pulsate

2 pressure on veins occludes them so that they appear most full distally

3 tendons have muscle tissue attached that can contract and act

4 ligamentous structures can be made to appear or disappear in different positions of joints.

Examination of the part

Before performing massage on either a model on whom you will practise or a patient whom you will treat you should examine the part on which you are going to work. In the case of a patient you will, of course, have carried out a complete examination and assessment so that you are aware of the problems which the patient presents.

Whether working on a model or a patient having arranged him or her as described above you should now examine the part you intend to massage.

LOOK at the skin state for dryness, oiliness, wetness, hairiness and completeness—thus you observe bruises, abrasions and lacera-tions. Look also at the state of subcutaneous tissues—is the skin emaciated or well padded and if the former, is it taut? Is there any oedema or excess reddening?

FEEL run your hand down the length of the part on every aspect. *Think* as you do so and be aware not only of the temperature of each area, the degree of muscle tension and joint posture but of any flinching as painful or ticklish areas are touched. Make mental notes so that problem areas can be approached with caution.

Ticklish subjects

People who are ticklish can be massaged without discomfort to them provided you observe the rules of always putting your hands in very firm contact as you start work and never lifting your hands off by 'trickling' i.e. by lifting your palms off first, then each phalanx, until only your finger tips are in contact.

You should also never move one hand component, especially fingers, in relation to one another once you have placed your hands in contact.

Light work tickles, so always perform the manipulations at the maximum depth tolerable by the model/patient and to produce the required result.

Chapter 2: The Massage Manipulations

The manipulations described in this chapter are:
- the effleurage/stroking manipulations
- the petrissage manipulations
- the friction manipulations
- the percussive (tapôtement) manipulations.

The effleurage/stroking manipulations

The word 'effleurage' means to stroke, and the manipulations in this group may be divided into:

1 Those in which the intention is primarily to assist venous and lymphatic drainage and in which the direction of the work is from distal to proximal—usually called effleurage.

2 Those in which the intention is primarily to obtain a sensory reaction either sedative or stimulative and in which direction is not important but is often from proximal to distal—usually called stroking.

In this book the words effleurage and stroking will apply to the above respective descriptions.

Effleurage

Effleurage is a *unidirectional* manipulation in which the operator's hand passes from distal to proximal with a depth compatible with the state of the tissues and the desired effect. Thus, the manipulation may start at one end and proceed to the proximal space, draining the part to be treated, e.g. finger tips to axilla, toes to groin, buttocks to axilla, neck to supraclavicular glands. The depth should be such as to push fluid onwards in the superficial vessels. This may be observed especially in the veins of the forearm. The manipulation is performed with the whole hand softly curved and relaxed to fit the part or with any part of the hand which fits the part. Both hands may be used together (Fig. 2.1) on opposite aspects of a part, or may follow one another (Fig. 2.2). Each hand may be used singly while the opposite hand supports the part in an appropriate position (Fig. 2.3). As the manipulation proceeds over the part, the hand(s) must change shape to maintain perfect contact.

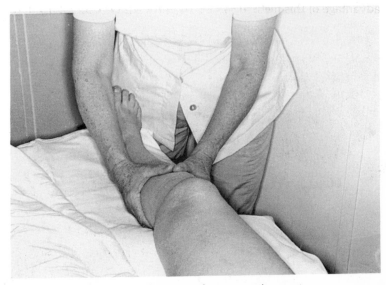

Fig. 2.1 Effleurage using both hands together on opposite aspects.

The stance of the operator is very important as these manipulations often proceed over a considerable length of the body, and it must be possible for the operator to transfer body weight to and fro. Walk standing (Fig. 1.2) is the usual stance adopted, with the weight being transferred from the rear to the forward foot accompanied, if need be, by either or both lifting of the heel of the rear foot, and flexion and extension of the knees and hips (Fig. 1.1). The arms will initially be flexed and become more extended especially at the elbows as the 'reach' is made. Integration of the arm and body movements must be obtained to ensure a smooth movement of the hand along the part; this is achieved if the arms stretch first followed by the body weight transfer. At the end of every line of effleurage there should be a small increase in depth (often called overpressure) and a slight pause (in the space) before the hand is lifted off with minimum flourish and returned to the distal part to start the next line of work. Some people advocate stroking the hand back to the start. The disadvantage of this method can be either a tickling effect if the return

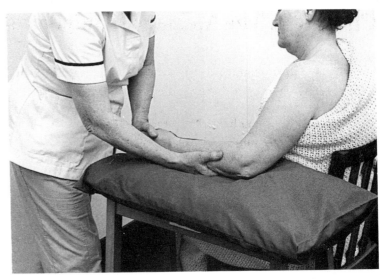

Fig. 2.3 Effleurage using one hand while the other hand supports.

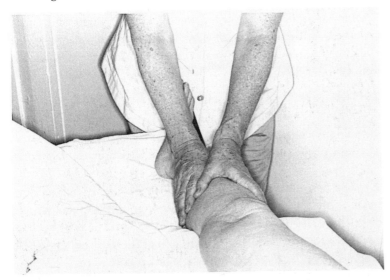

Fig. 2.2 Effleurage using both hands together following one another.

stroke is too light or a feeling of downdrag if the return stroke is too deep.

When the whole hand is used for effleurage, it does not maintain equal contact over its whole surface and should be placed obliquely on the skin so that the leading edge is the 'C' formed by the thumb to forefinger cleft. This edge is formed by the lateral border of the forefinger and the medial border of the thumb linked by the adjacent web; *however*, the main pressure is exerted by the 'C' formed by the lateral border of the thumb, the thenar eminence, the hypothenar eminence and the little finger. The pressure is graded from the index to little fingers and adjacent parts of the palm so that the hand operates in the manner of a ski.

If the pressure is exerted by the leading edge, it can be uncomfortable or jerky, or can cause sticking. Lack of control of the modulation of the pressure as the hand proceeds up the part is more usually caused by:

either

standing too near the finish of the stroke (step back to cure this),
or

by failing to synchronize the arm movements with the weight transfer (see page 9).

Stroking

Stroking is a unidirectional manipulation in which the operator's hand passes, usually, from proximal to distal down the length of the tissues at a depth and speed compatible with the required effect, but direction of the stroke may be varied to give greater comfort.

The stroke should start with firm contact (try not to trickle your fingers on) and finish with a smooth lift off of your hands. The hands may be positioned obliquely or so that the heel travels first, but can adjust its position down the length of the part so that comfortable contact is maintained.

The slower strokes are more sedative. Try a speed of one stroke per five seconds.

The faster strokes are more stimulating. Try a speed of four strokes every five seconds, i.e. four times faster.

Obviously greater depth can be achieved at the slower rate, but the need for sedative effects may limit your depth when pain and muscle spasm prevent firmer contact. If this is so, the depth is increased as relaxation occurs and pain diminishes but the tempo should still be maintained. The faster stroking is often used to complete a more stimulating massage.

The whole area under treatment should be covered by a sequence of strokes. Stroking may be performed using:

1 one hand—usually on a narrow area
2 two hands simultaneously—one each side on a broad area—be careful not to pull on the part (Fig. 1.1)
3 right and left hands following one another on a narrow area
4 thumb(s) or fingers(s) on confined areas one-handed, two-handed or alternately
5 a technique called 'thousand hands' in which one hand performs a short stroke, the second hand does the same overlapping the first, and the hands pass over one another to gain contact as the manipulation proceeds down the length of the part under treatment.

The petrissage manipulation

Petrissage manipulations are those in which the soft tissues (mainly muscles) are compressed either against underlying bone or against themselves. They are divided into:

• **kneading manipulations**—when the tissues are compressed against the underlying structures
• **picking up manipulations**—when the tissues are compressed then lifted and squeezed
• **wringing manipulations**—when the tissues are lifted and squeezed by alternating hand pressure
• **rolling manipulations**—when the tissues are lifted and rolled between the fingers and thumbs as in skin rolling or muscle rolling
• **shaking manipulations**—when the tissues are lifted and shaken from side to side.

Kneading

Kneading is a circular manipulation performed so that the skin and subcutaneous tissues are moved in a circular manner on the underlying structures. The manipulation may be performed with the palmar aspect of the whole hand, with the palm only, with all the fingers, with the pads or tips of the thumb or of the fingers. Whatever the area used, a circle is described by the part of your hand in contact, with pressure on the upward part of the circle but only for a small segment. The actual range or number of degrees for which pressure is exerted varies with the part treated.

On flat areas, e.g. the back, the pressure with the right hand is from 8 o'clock to 11 o'clock with that hand circling clockwise. The left hand circles anti-clockwise and exerts pressure from 4 o'clock to 1 o'clock (Fig. 2.4). On the limbs, the pressure is exerted from 6 o'clock to 9 o'clock with the right hand and from 6 o'clock to 3 o'clock with the left hand. On the non-pressure phase of the circle the hand maintains contact but glides on to the next area of skin a small enough distance to allow the next circle to cover at least half the previous area. The right hand moving clockwise will slide downwards from 4 o'clock, while the left hand will glide downwards from 8 o'clock (Fig. 2.4). Great care must be taken to transmit the required pressure to get the necessary depth through the whole hand and not just the heel of the hand. This is effected by correct foot position and body position giving a correct relationship to the part under treatment, plus integrated flexion of hips, shoulders and elbows to transfer and use body weight. In performing all kneading manipulations use walk standing so that your body weight can move easily from one foot to the other.

Kneading may be performed with:

1 the whole hand—whole hand kneading (Fig. 2.5)
2 the palm only—palmar kneading (Fig. 2.6)
3 the fingers only—
   (a) flat finger kneading (Fig. 2.7)
   (b) finger pad kneading (Fig. 2.8)
   (c) finger tip kneading (Fig. 2.9)
4 the thumb—
   (a) thumb pad kneading (Fig. 2.10)
   (b) thumb tip kneading (Fig. 2.11)
5 both hands when one is superimposed on the other—superimposed (reinforced) kneading (Fig. 2.12)

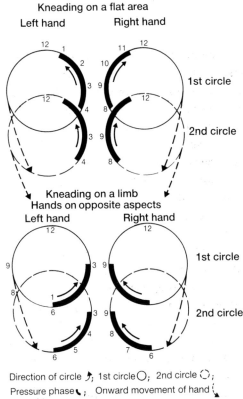

Kneading on a flat area
Left hand   Right hand

1st circle

2nd circle

Kneading on a limb
Hands on opposite aspects
Left hand   Right hand

1st circle

2nd circle

Direction of circle ↗; 1st circle ◯; 2nd circle ◌;
Pressure phase ◖; Onward movement of hand ↙

Fig. 2.4 Kneading: the right hand works clockwise and the left hand anticlockwise. Pressure is exerted for the shaded part of the circle only. a, on a flat area (the back) b, on a round area (the limbs). The hands move on at the down-pointing arrows.

In the case of the first four options, the manipulation may be performed:

- single-handed (Fig. 2.13)
- double-handed—alternately (Fig. 2.5)
          simultaneously (Fig. 2.11)

The choice is dictated to some extent by the size of the part under treatment and by the state of the tissues. For example, superimposed kneading has considerable depth and is used on the back and gluteal regions, thumb and finger tip kneading is used on narrow muscle groups such as the interossei or peronei, *but* subjects with very mobile skins may not be suitable for simultaneous double handed kneading as it is too easy to perform a large range manipulation and cause the subject to slide up and down on the bed. This is especially so when working on the back with the subject in prone lying.

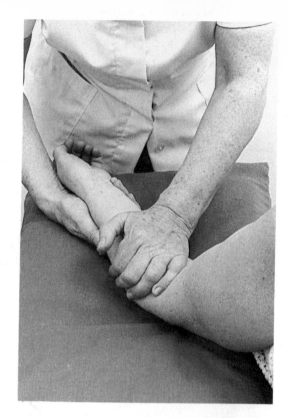

Fig. 2.6 Kneading with the palm only—palmar kneading.

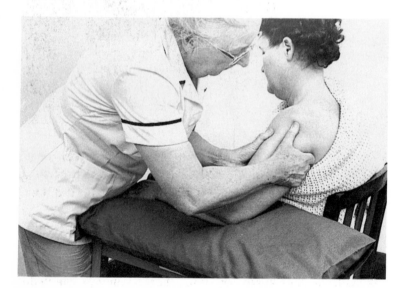

Fig. 2.5 Kneading: using the whole palmar aspect of the hand.

Performance

Stand in walk standing.

1 Whole hand kneading—place your hand obliquely to the long axis of the part and maintain full contact using all of the palmar surface to perform the manipulation (Fig. 2.5).

2 Palmar kneading—use only the palm of your hand and allow your fingers and thumb to relax off-contact with the subject. Great depth can be gained using the palm so take care not to dig in with the bony prominences of the carpus (Fig. 2.6).

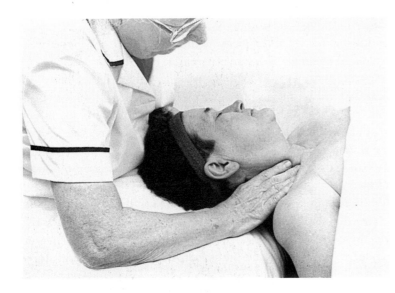

Fig. 2.7 Flat finger kneading.

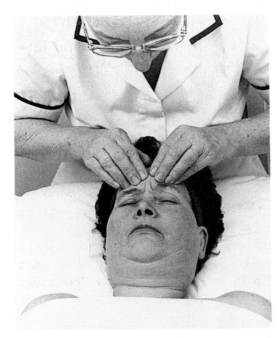

Fig. 2.8 Finger pad kneading.

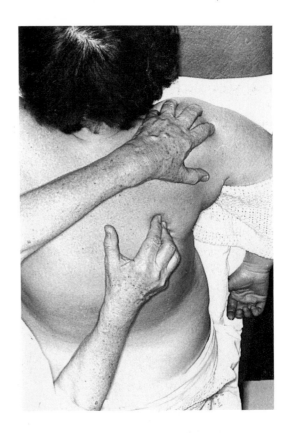

Fig. 2.9 Finger tip kneading.

3 (a) Flat finger kneading is performed with the palmar surfaces of the 2nd to 5th digits while the palm and thumb remain off-contact. It is often used to work on less muscular or poorly padded areas (Fig. 2.7).

(b) Finger pad kneading is performed with the finger pads either individually, when index on middle fingers are more commonly used, or with several finger pads together to provide a linear contact (Fig. 2.8). The little finger may be too short on most people so the index, middle and ring fingers are bent sufficiently to allow the pads to create a contact line. These manipulations are often used round joints and along the line of ligaments and in treating scars.

(c) Finger tip kneading is performed in the same way as finger pad kneading but using only the tip of the pad, taking care to keep your nails off-contact (Fig. 2.9). Narrow, linear areas are dealt with using several finger tips, and one finger tip should be used on small structures or to work on painful areas when the patient will tolerate only very small contact and no movement of the part.

4 (a) Thumb kneading is performed with the thumb pads. The size of the area to be treated dictates the amount of the pad which is in contact with the subject's skin. On the larger areas, such as the forearm, back and leg, the whole pad is used (Fig. 2.10). The manipulation is usually performed by resting your fingers on the opposite side of the limbs or more laterally on the back, but when working on the face, or in the presence of any contra-indications the fingers should not rest on the subject. The skin and subcutaneous tissues should be moved on the underlying tissues so as to produce a wrinkle on the outer sides of the working thumb (Fig. 2.10). Mobile, well-padded skin allows a greater range circle to be performed.

Note also the position of the working and resting thumbs. Both lie at an angle to the long axis of the limb, the resting thumb in position ready to start the next circle, while the working thumb maintains the same angle but describes a circle. In other words, the thumb angles to the limb or part only change to accommodate the size of the part and the thumb should never slide into adduction.

The working thumb will almost invariably have to pass the resting thumb and should do so by slipping past its tip in contact. If the thumb is lifted to move on, then a 'cat walking' effect is produced, the length of the thumb contact is lost and the pressure of the manipulation will be more likely to be too deep, uneven and less effective.

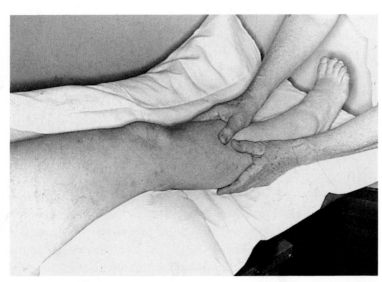

Fig. 2.10   Thumb pad kneading.

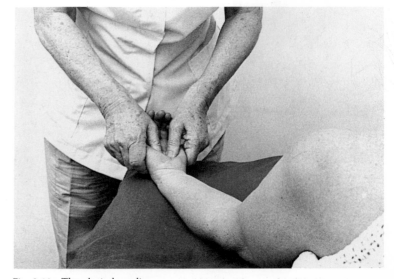

Fig. 2.11   Thumb tip kneading.

(b) Thumb tip kneading is performed more frequently with the side of the thumb tip and is useful when the part to be treated has a long, narrow shape—as the interosseus spaces. Your fingers act as counter supports on the opposite aspect of the part and your thumb should lie in adduction so that your lateral thumb tip is in contact without involving your nail (Fig. 5.10).

5 Superimposed (re-inforced) kneading. This type of kneading can be very deep and is usually performed when greater depth is required. The contact hand is rested fully on the part, the superimposed hand rests on top of it either obliquely across when working on the opposite side of the body (Fig. 2.12) or palm over fingers as in Fig. 6.9 when working on the adjacent side of the body. The upper hand must not exert such constant pressure that the kneading by the under hand is distorted. Both hands work together. The body movements of the operator are a forward and back-ward sway from the feet, to enchance depth, but control must be exerted to prevent the circle of the kneading developing a sharp point at the moment of maximum pressure combined with the movement of the hands as they perform the most distant part of the circle.

Picking up

Picking up is a manipulation in which the tissues are compressed against underlying bone, then lifted, squeezed and released. The manipulation is more usually performed singlehanded with the thumb and thenar eminence as one component and the medial two or three fingers and hypothenar eminence as the other component of the grasp. The thumb must be opposed and abducted and the degree of these two movements will produce:

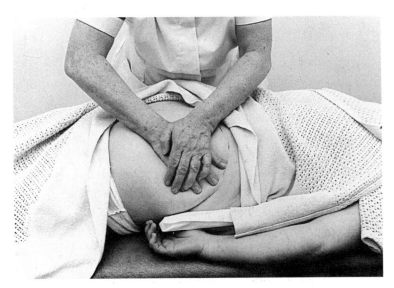

Fig. 2.12 Superimposed (re-inforced) kneading.

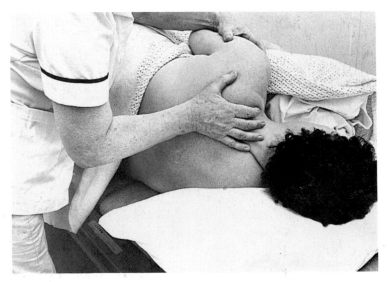

Fig. 2.13 Single-handed kneading.

either a 'C' shaped grasp (Fig. 2.14) which is wider on larger areas, **or** a 'V' shaped grasp (Fig. 2.15) which is narrower on areas of lesser bulk.

The cleft between the thumb and index finger should always be in contact with the subject's skin otherwise a pinching effect is produced and depth is lost.

As body weight transfer is important, walk standing is the stance required.

Picking up should be performed with your arms held in slight abduction and with semi-flexed elbows. The wrists are always used initially extended and are more extended as the grasp is effected. Your wrists should never be flexed as this will cause you to pivot on your thumb and finger tips with a screwing action.

Place your hand on the part so that the thumb cleft lies across the centre line of the muscle bulk with your thumb and thenar

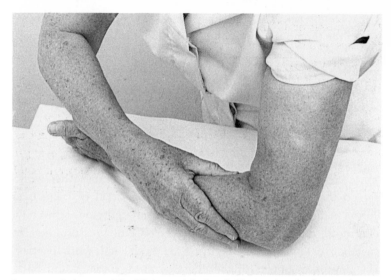

Fig. 2.15   Picking up. The 'V' shape of the hand. (Practise on own forearm.)

eminence disposed on one side and your medial two or three fingers and hypothenar eminence on the other side. Exert compression by transferring your body weight from your feet through your forearm and to the whole hand. Count this as ONE. Then immediately grasp, using the two grasp components equally so that your wrist extends more but do not further flex any part of your thumb and fingers. This exerts a squeeze and a simultaneous lift of the tissues will occur. Count this as TWO. Release your grasp—count this as THREE. Your body weight should still be forward, but as you move your relaxed hand on to the next part maintaining the current conformation, take your body weight back again to your starting position. Count this as FOUR. Thus the body weight movement is:

• forward on the count ONE
• backward on the count FOUR

while the hand:

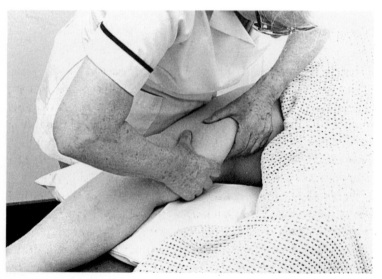

Fig. 2.14   Picking up. The 'C' shape of the hand. Also shows double handed, alternate work.

- compresses on ONE
- grasps on TWO (lift occurs)
- releases on THREE
- moves on FOUR

Learning this combination of movements is one of the more difficult tasks in massage training. Practise first with each hand working backward, down the length of a muscle (Fig. 2.14) or up the length of a muscle. Then try travelling in the reverse direction on the longer muscle masses as in the lower limb, leading up to working one hand travelling backwards as the other hand travels forwards at such a distance so that your fingers and thumbs never touch but the muscle is constantly lifted (Fig. 2.15).

Alternatively, on larger muscle masses such as the anterior aspect of the thigh, your two hands may work as one unit spanning the muscle. Your hands lie so that the thumb of the first hand lies alongside the index finger of the second hand. The thumb of this second hand lies under the heel and alongside the hypothenar eminence of the first hand (Fig. 2.16). The compression is performed by both your hands. The grasp is performed by radial extension of both wrists so that the tissues are lifted and squeezed between the medial part of the palms and medial three fingers of both hands. The tissues are released, and your hands move backwards as one unit for one third of their length on to a new area.

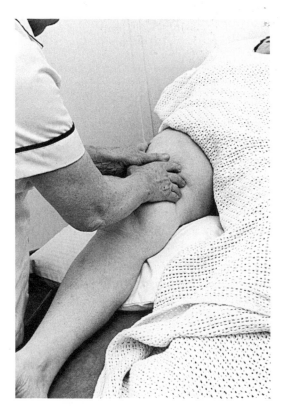

Fig. 2.16 Picking up. Double handed simultaneous work.

Wringing

Wringing is a manipulation in which the tissues are compressed against the underlying structures prior to lifting them, as in picking up. Then, instead of squeezing the tissues, you pull gently towards yourself with the fingers of one hand while the thumb of your other hand pushes gently in the opposite direction. The tissues are kept elevated and passed from hand to hand by moving the non-pressing component of each hand in turn along the tissues (Fig. 2.17a).

The smaller the tissue, the more the tips of your thumbs and fingers are used, and your arms are more adducted and wrists lifted to be more alongside one another. If your arms are abducted and your wrists and forearms lie more parallel with the long axis of the tissues then the bigger manipulation can be performed. When the tissue is very small, as in the case of the tendocalcaneus, the manipulation is performed between your thumbs and finger tips as in

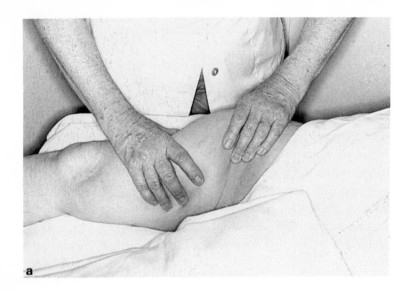

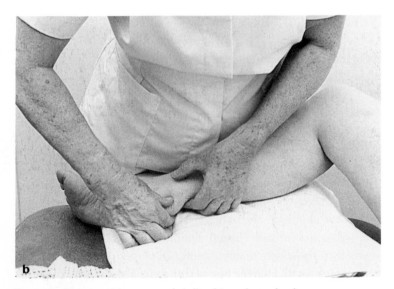

Fig. 2.17 Wringing: (a) on a muscle belly; (b) on the tendocalcaneous.

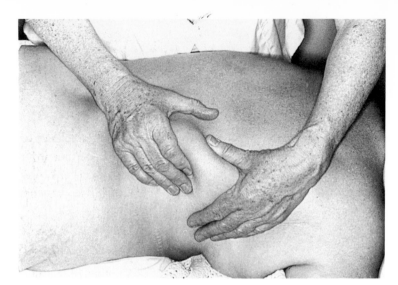

Fig. 2.18 Wringing on superficial tissues.

Fig. 2.17b. There is an intermediate manner of performance on small muscle groups such as the upper limb muscles. Greater length of your finger pads is used with your thumbs turned so that a greater length of your thumb pad is available on the other side of the muscle tissue. The manipulation may also be performed as a skin wringing, an alternative to skin rolling when only the superficial tissues are lifted and wrung (Fig. 2.18).

Rolling manipulations

The most common rolling manipulation is skin rolling, but muscles may also be rolled.

Skin rolling

Skin rolling is a manipulation in which the skin is lifted and rolled between the thumbs and fingers of the two hands. The manipulation

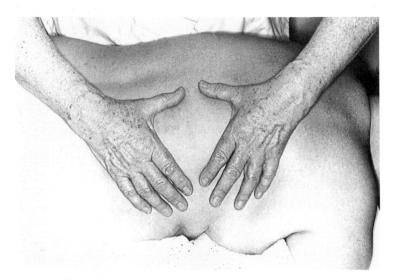

Fig. 2.19 Skin rolling—start.

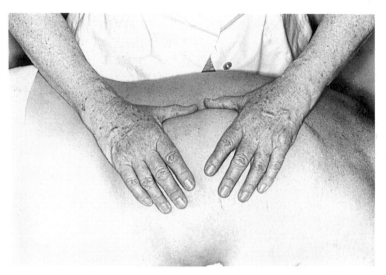

Fig. 2.20 Skin rolling—pull back.

is most often performed on the back, abdomen and thighs but it is also used round superficial joints such as the knee, and in modified form on scar tissue which is shortening and thickening.

Stand in walk standing at the side of the area to be treated and facing across it. Place both hands on the surface of the area more distal from you so that your palms are fully in contact, with your thumb tips touching and parallel to the long axis of the part. Your thumbs should be abducted to such an extent that your index fingers do not touch and indeed should have a space between them (Fig. 2.19).

Maintain full palmar contact and pull your hands backwards towards yourself, without changing their shape and with sufficient pressure to pull the underlying skin (Fig. 2.20). Next, apply pressure with your thumbs as you adduct and oppose them with some depth so that they remain in line with each other but the skin is pushed in a roll towards the fingers (Fig. 2.21). Almost simultaneously, your

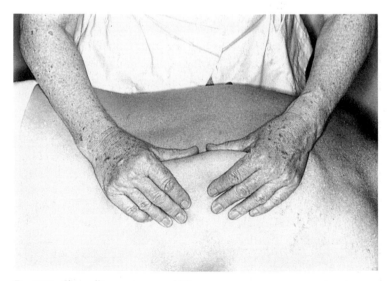

Fig. 2.21 Skin rolling—squeeze and lift.

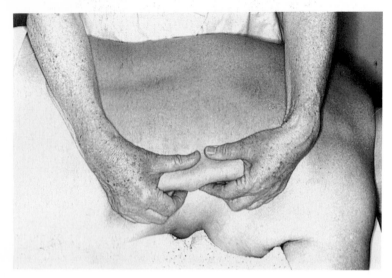

Fig. 2.22 Skin rolling—roll.

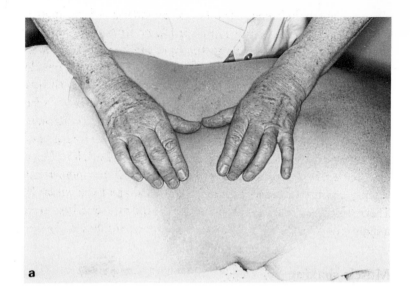

palms should gradually lift off the skin but your finger tips should remain in contact. Now roll your thumbs forwards still maintaining the roll of skin in your grasp and the skin will roll against your fingers. Your wrists should be flexed and ulnar deviated as this occurs, so that the skin is folded over on top of your fingers (Fig. 2.22).

Try not to 'creep' your fingers as you roll as this can tickle. On adherent skins the skin will only lift slightly and the length of the rolling action must be shortened. The model shown in Figs 2.19—2.22 had very mobile skin and half the width of the back could be treated at once. For adherent skin two or three lines of work should be done instead of the one line shown in Figs 2.19—2.22.

Muscle rolling

Muscle rolling is performed by working across the muscle fibres and along the long axis of muscles. You should be in walk standing to

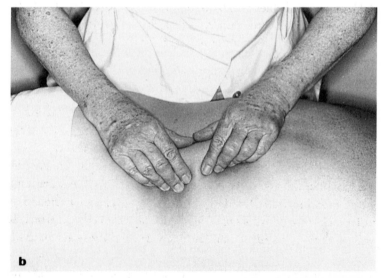

Fig. 2.23 Muscle rolling: (a) Push with the flat thumbs. (b) Pull back with the finger tips.

allow weight transference. The lateral boundaries of the muscle should be palpated, then your thumbs placed tip to tip along one border with your fingers along the opposite border (Fig. 2.23). Apply a little pressure with both components so that the muscle bulges slightly between your thumbs and fingers. Then push first with your thumbs and release the pressure simultaneously with the fingers which move to an adjacent area (Fig. 2.23a). Rapidly reverse, pressing with the fingers and releasing the pressure of your thumbs which also move to an adjacent area (Fig. 2.23b). It is often a more effective and comfortable manipulation if the pressure is slightly down into the muscle mass than back and forth across it. This manipulation can be performed slowly and deliberately to exert a slight stretch or faster so that there is stimulation to the circulation.

Muscle shaking

All long muscle bellies may be shaken and the manipulation may be performed on the larger muscles such as biceps, triceps, the quadriceps and also on the small muscles of the thenar and hypothenar eminences.

The manipulation is one in which:

For longer muscles the length of your thumb should be placed on one side of the muscle belly and all your fingers placed on the other side of the muscle belly. Your palm should be off-contact (Fig. 2.24). Your hand is then rapidly shaken from side to side as you traverse the length of the muscle belly avoiding contact with the underlying bone. Stand in walk standing so that your weight is transferred as you work from proximal to distal on the muscle belly. The muscle will be 'thrown' rapidly from side to side and feels very invigorated.

For very small muscles, the tip of your thumb should be placed on one side, and an appropriate number of finger tips placed on the

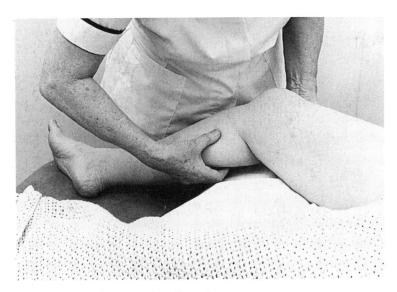

Fig. 2.24   Muscle shaking on the calf muscles.

other side of the muscle belly, and the shaking movement described above is performed.

The friction manipulations

Frictions are small range, deep manipulations performed on specific anatomical structures with the tips of the fingers or thumbs. No other part of the practitioner's hand must rest on the part. There are two types of frictions:
- circular
- transverse.

Circular frictions

Circular frictions are performed with the finger tips. The structure to be treated should be identified by careful palpation and the finger

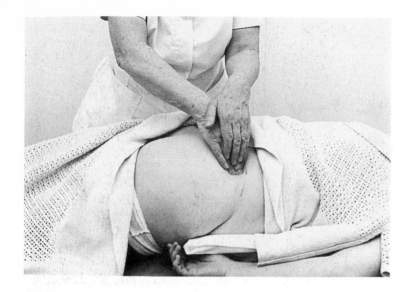

Fig. 2.25 Circular frictions to the attachments on the iliac crest.

tip(s) placed so that they cover the area. The rest of the hand is kept off-contact. Pressure is applied and a small, stationary manipulation is performed, in a circular manner and at gradually increasing depth for three or four circles. The pressure is released and the manipulation is repeated. One hand may re-inforce the other on deeper structures. The manipulation can be used over ligaments and myofascial junctions (Fig. 2.25).

Transverse frictions

Transverse frictions were advocated by Dr J. Cyriax in 1941 for treatment of tendon, ligament, myofascial junctions and muscles. The manipulation is performed with:
either the thumb tip
or the finger tip of the index finger sometimes reinforced by placing the tip of the middle finger on top of the index finger nail (Fig. 2.26)

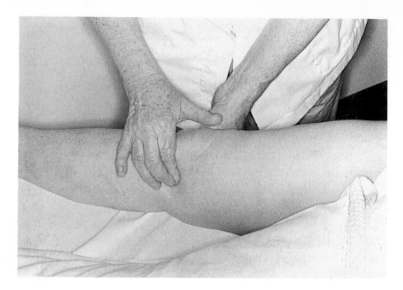

Fig. 2.26 Transverse friction to the medial ligament of the knee.

or by the middle finger reinforced by placing the index finger on top of the middle finger nail (more useful when the hand is curved round a limb)
or by two finger tips when a long structure is affected (such as a tendon)
or by the opposed fingers and thumb on structures which can be grasped e.g. tendocalcaneous.

Identify the structure to be treated, and place your fingers across the longitudinal axis of the structure i.e. across the length of the collagen fibres (Figs. 2.26, 2.27, 2.28, 2.29, 2.30).

Now perform the friction by moving your digit and the model's skin as one, keeping your digit, hand and forearm in a line parallel to the movement to be performed. Do not flex and extend only your digit or wrist. Learn to use both hands so that you lessen your own fatigue. Try to use a movement from your upper arm, trunk or feet

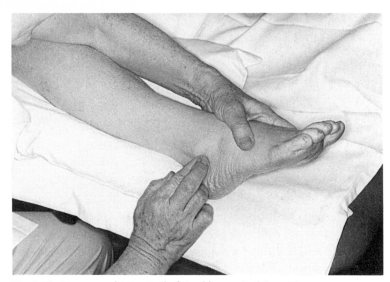

Fig. 2.27 Transverse friction to the lateral ligament of the ankle.

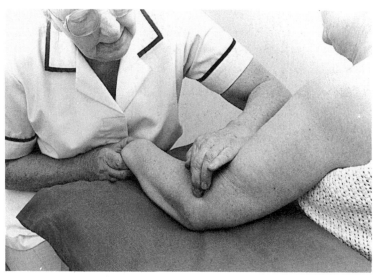

Fig. 2.29 Transverse friction to the common extensor tendon.

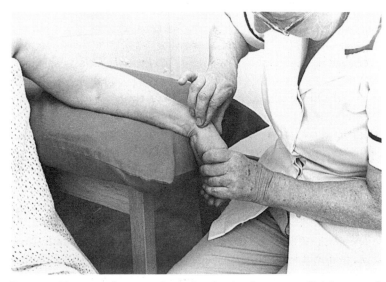

Fig. 2.28 Transverse friction to the tendon sheaths of extensor pollicis longus and abductor pollicis longus.

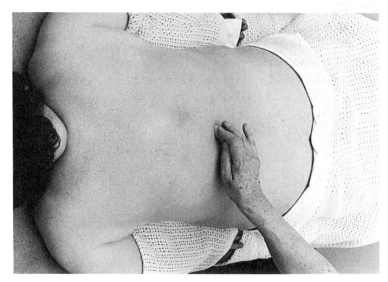

Fig. 2.30 Transverse friction to supraspinous ligament.

so that you achieve greater power with less fatigue. Either sit down or stand in walk standing.

Start to move your fingers forwards and backwards across the structure under treatment with sufficient sweep to produce separation of the fibres at a depth to engage the affected tissue rather than at the patient's tolerance. He or she should be warned that the treatment may be painful, but that numbness may supervene as it progresses. The movement must not take place between your fingers and the model's skin, but between the affected structure and the overlying tissues.

The model's skin must be dry to ensure your fingers do not slip. If necessary, apply either spirit or a wisp of cotton wool to the part. The wool is kept in position during the treatment. With these precautions blistering should not occur, but transient redness or slight bruising in adipose tissue may arise.

Maintain the friction for five to ten minutes but the area should be examined at intervals to check that bruising is not occurring nor the skin blistering.

Keep tendons taut by putting them on the stretch (Figs. 2.28 and 2.29), but keep muscles relaxed, by positioning the model so that the part and the attachments of the muscle are approximated during treatment.

Tapôtement or percussive manipulations

The percussive manipulations are those in which the treated part is struck soft blows with the hands. They are performed either to assist evacuation from hollow organs, or to stimulate either skin or muscle reflexes. Stand in walk standing and try practising on a pillow or a padded couch, except for vibrations which may be practised on a partly filled hot water bag.

The manipulations are:

1 clapping
2 hacking
3 vibrations (shakings)
4 beating
5 pounding
6 tapping.

Clapping

Clapping (Figs 2.31, 2.32 and 2.33) is a manipulation in which the whole palmar aspect of the hand is used to strike the body part. The hand is, however, cupped in such a manner that the centre of the hand does not touch the part, but is hollowed. The fingers are slightly flexed, more so at the metacarpophalangeal joints of the index, middle and ring fingers. The thumb is adducted so that it lies just under the index finger and adjacent palm. The hand must be kept in this posture but as relaxed as possible. The wrists should be used to create the difference between striking a hollow sounding blow and a slightly sharper blow. (Slapping sounds very sharp.) The former will have the depth to cause 'jarring' and is used to evacuate hollow organs. The latter is for skin stimulation.

The difference is brought about by the arm movements performed and the effects they have on the hands. The percussive effect is achieved when the heel of the hand is lifted from the part more than the finger tips. The wrist is thus flexed (Fig. 2.31). This movement is brought about by lifting the arm into abduction (beer drinking action when using a tankard) and allowing it to drop. The velocity of the drop (not the height) creates the depth of the work.

This deeper manipulation is usually performed with the skin lightly covered by a sheet, thin blanket or a single layer of the patient's clothing (Fig. 2.32).

The more stimulating manipulation is also brought about by arm abduction, but with the finger tips raised from the body part without increasing the wrist flexion. In other words the whole hand is raised. The 'strike' is brought about by actively lowering the arm

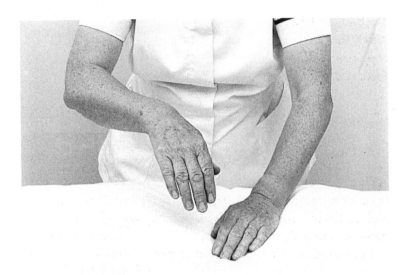

Fig. 2.31 Practising percussive clapping on a pillow.

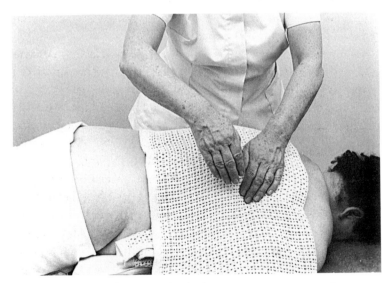

Fig. 2.32 Percussive clapping on the chest.

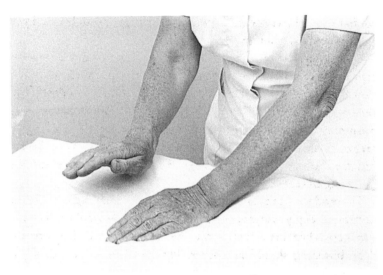

Fig. 2.33 Practising skin stimulating clapping on a pillow.

(Fig. 2.33). The tempo of the action should be slower to obtain greater depth, and faster for skin stimulation.

Hacking

Hacking is a manipulation in which the skin is struck using the back of the tips of the three medial fingers. A correct performance is dependent on:
- the initial posture of the whole of the operator's arms and hands with good wrist extension
- a good range of pronation and supination of the radio-ulnar joints.

The only movement required is that of pronation and supination. The elbows MUST NOT flex and extend. The hands are held at a small distance apart so that as they rotate alternately, they just clear one another. The arms are in slight abduction, the elbows are flexed to a right angle with the forearms held parallel with the model's skin

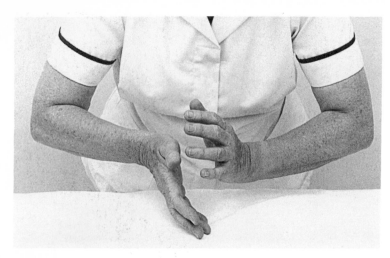

Fig. 2.34 Practising hacking on a pillow.

and far enough above it to allow only the backs of the little, ring and middle fingers to touch when the forearm is in supination. The wrists are well extended to about 50° (Fig. 2.34).

NB This manipulation cannot be performed properly with less than 50° extension of the wrists. The fingers are in relaxed flexion, i.e. the posture the relaxed hand adopts spontaneously, and are separated.

Experiment by resting the finger tips of your hands on each other with your little finger resting on the model's skin. Then, slightly separate the finger tips—less than 1.5 cm, and check to see if pronation and supination are alternately possible without your finger tips touching those of the other hand.

The 'strike' is modified by the vigour applied to the rotatory movement. A very light hacking produces a susurration, whereas vigorous hacking should sound like a sharp striking noise. Initially, try a slow rate of 10 strikes per five seconds with each hand, then work up to a fast rate of 20—30 strikes per five seconds with each

hand. Single strikes can achieve great depth and can be used to obtain reflex contractions of muscle. Slow, deep hacking may produce mechanical effects on hollow organs. All hacking, but especially fast work, produces effects on the skin circulation, and appropriate subjects demonstrate this by producing distinct erythema (reddening) of the skin at the points of strike.

Vibrations

Vibrations are often wrongly called shakings. The difference is that a vibration involves a movement in which the tissues are pressed and released using an up and down motion. In shaking, the movement on the model is sideways, and involves rapid radial and ulnar deviation of your wrists.

Vibrations may be fine or very coarse and demonstrate best on a partly filled rubber hot water bag or on the abdomen (Fig. 2.35), though the more common use is on the chest.

Vibrations may be performed with the whole hand, or the finger tips. Practise with your hand stationary or slide backwards and forwards on the area. They are best practised by placing the whole hand on a partly filled hot water bag with the arm outstretched, and oscillating your whole hand into rapid and minute wrist flexion and extension. The movement is sustained from the shoulder and can be observed to occur spontaneously in some people if the arms are outstretched.

Beating

Beating is a much less used manipulation in which the loosely clenched fist is used for the 'strike'. Its value lies in that the hand is made smaller, but is used as in clapping.

The fingers are flexed at the metacarpophalangeal and proximal interphalangeal joints, but extended at the distal interphalangeal

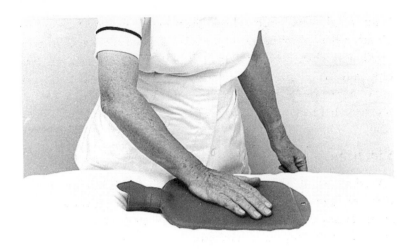

a

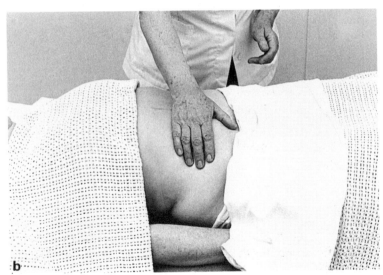

b

Fig. 2.35 Practising vibrations on: (a) a rubber water bag; (b) the abdomen.

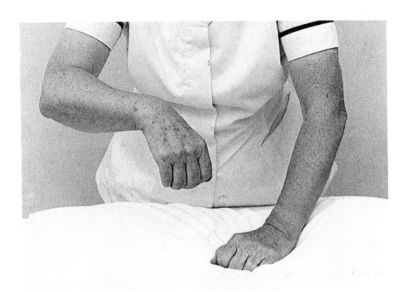

Fig. 2.36 Practising beating on a pillow.

joints so that there is a flat surface composed of the backs of the two distal phalanges and the margin of the palmar surface of the palm. The thumb is kept flat against the lateral part of the flexed hand. The most important part of the operator's action is to raise the whole arm into abduction and allow the wrist to droop (Fig. 2.36) in relaxation. The arm is allowed to drop and strike the part. The speed to attain is six strikes per 10 seconds.

Pounding

Pounding is a less used manipulation but also has value in that it is a form of hacking done with a loosely clenched fist.

The fingers are loosely flexed at all the joints and the thumb lies flat on the lateral side of the hand in halfway position between adduction and flexion. The action is exactly that of hacking, i.e.

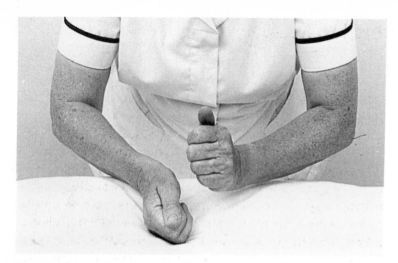

Fig. 2.37   Practising pounding on a pillow.

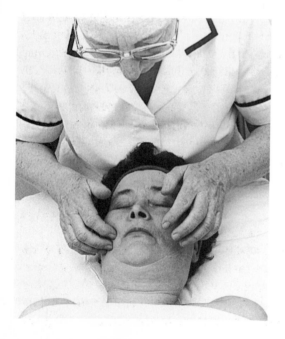

Fig. 2.38   Tapping on the face.

pronation and supination of the semi-flexed forearms so that the 'strike' is with the knuckles of the little finger (Fig. 2.37). The rate of 'strike' is slightly slower than in hacking.

Tapping

Tapping is performed with the tips of the finger pads and is used on very small areas such as the face (Fig. 2.38). The hand is held relaxed over the area to be treated and the fingers tap at a depth to produce a slightly hollow sound. The index, middle and ring fingers may be used together or in any smaller number, or these three fingers may be used singly in sequence. Both forms of tapping are seen in restless or irritated people who tap chair arms.

Chapter 3: Effects of and Contra-indications for Massage

The effects of massage

The effects of massage are now more recognized in an intellectual way, but for centuries the animal kingdom has used 'rubbing' of different types to deal with the discomforts of living. We have all observed domesticated animals 'licking' and so 'stroking' wounded areas, and puppies and kittens being licked to facilitate digestive functions.

Some primates also rub each other to assist toleration of/and relief of disorder. Every one of us has been rubbed or patted in infancy to assist voiding of wind and also to comfort and induce sleep in the fretful. Most of us will have held and then rubbed our bumps and painful areas such as disordered joints and muscles.

Massage has effects which can be described under the following main headings:

1 mechanical
2 physiological, subdivided into:
   (a) circulatory
   (b) neurological
   (c) dermal.

Mechanical effects

The squeezing, compressive and pushing components of the massage manipulation bring about drainage of venous blood and lymph. The drainage of venous blood can be observed if a dependent hand in which the superficial veins are easily observed, is stroked firmly.

The soft walled veins are compressed and the blood within them flows onward or centripetally. Its return is stopped by the presence of valves which prevent backflow and by the blood behind waiting to take its place. Lymph vessels are also thin walled and affected in the same way. All the minute drainage vessels must be equally affected so that as blood and lymph flows onwards more rapidly due to the massage the replacing blood moves more quickly. In this way the drainage of treated tissues is enhanced allowing fresh blood an unimpeded flow.

Mobilization of the tissues treated also occurs as they are moved or move on one another. It is noticeable that many of the manipulations cause slight stretch, thus maintaining elasticity and regaining mobility where tissues are tending to adhere within themselves or to adjacent or surrounding tissues. This mobilizing effect in enhanced by the fresh blood supply which will cause increased warmth of the part. Static blood is cooler than moving blood, and a sluggish circulation is usually accompanied by reduced temperature of the tissues involved. Firmer stretching manipulations are likely to stretch adhesions and, some authorities claim, break them down. Envisage this not as snapping of a strand of silk, but as re-absorption of the forming scar tissue which is creating the adhesions; and of lengthening effects on the adhering and scar tissue.

The percussive manipulations performed over the lungs, have the mechanical effect of jerking adherent mucous free from the bronchial tree and, aided by gravity, assisting the removal of sputum towards the upper respiratory passages. The jarring effect and the vibratory effect probably cause some mixing of respiratory gases, while vibrations performed on the distended, wind-laden abdomen cause movement of the wind and relief of discomfort, whether in the infant after a feed, or patients in the post-operative abdominal recovery stage.

Physiological effects

On the circulation

Physiological effects on the circulation arise from the improved drainage as the drained blood and lymph will remove metabolites. The pressure of the massage manipulations increases the interstitial pressure and thus aids absorption of tissue fluid across the capillary walls. The fresh blood flowing in to the part will improve its metabolism as the oxygen and food supply to the part is enhanced.

Cutaneous circulatory responses also occur in the following order:

1 A transient white line appears in response to light pressure and is the result of an initial capillary constriction.

2 Because the tissues are slightly traumatized by most massage manipulations and more so by those such as skin rolling and the percussive manipulations, a histamine-related substance is released. Histamine is stored in mast cells in the connective tissues, and in the basophil cells and platelets of blood, all of which may be disturbed or traumatized by the various massage manipulations. The effect of release of this substance is the triple response which follows. It involves three reactions which follow each other rapidly. A red line appears and is caused by dilatation of the minute blood vessels independent of the somatic supply of the skin area. A flare of redness often described as a 'flush' then appears around the area and is due to a widespread dilatation of skin arterioles. This is brought about by the axon reflex. The third feature of the triple response is slight swelling usually described as a wheal. The increased permeability of the capillary walls allows escape of more tissue fluid so that the area becomes slightly swollen. This fluid is almost identical with lymph.

On the nervous system

Physiological effects on the nervous system are counter-irritant, inhibitory and excitatory. The counter-irritant effect occurs, for example, when frictions are applied and a competing pain produced by the massage manipulation is given priority over the painful stimulus. The competition for recognition by the two stimuli—the old and new, probably occurs at the synapses in the central nervous system. Inhibitory effects are:

either direct when constant repetition of the same, slow, soothing manipulation brings about accommodation by raising the threshold of perception

or indirect when the resultant lessened flow of stimuli from the sensory nerve endings in the treated area reduces the inflow to the motor neurones of the spinal cord.

Muscle tone is thus reduced and muscle spasm will be relieved. Pain will also consequently be relieved.

Excitation can have a direct effect when stimulation of skin receptors or stretch of muscle spindles reflexly increases the muscle tone. The other reflex responses which may occur are stimulation of the sweat glands and increased heart rate.

On the skin

The skin itself shows physiological effects in addition to those already described. The constant passage of the hands over the skin will remove dead surface cells and allow the sweat glands, the hair follicles and the sebaceous glands to be free of obstruction and to function better. Combined with the improved circulation which these structures have from massage, the noticeable effect is often a more lubricated appearance and feeling of the skin. This is especially noticeable when desquamation is a problem.

Psychological effects are best evinced when a patient says following massage 'That feels better.' Massage may induce a feeling of well-being in the area treated, it relieves pain, so reducing fear, and helps to reassure patients that painful and damaged parts can be touched and moved.

In addition massage gives the comfort provided by the caring touch of one human being on another. and

Contra-indications

Massage is contra-indicated in the following circumstances:
1 skin disorders which would be irritated by either increase in warmth of the part or by the lubricants which might be used e.g. eczema.
When superficial infections are suppurating.
2 in the presence of malignant tumours
3 early bruising—though at about the fourth day massage will be of use in treating a haematoma
4 in the presence of recent, unhealed scars or open wounds
5 adjacent to recent fracture sites and especially at the elbow or mid-thigh
6 over joints or other tissues which are acutely inflamed especially joints with tubercular infections.

In a Seperate page

Chapter 4: Massage to the Upper Limb

The whole upper limb is usually treated as one unit. It is so much smaller than the lower limb that it is possible to work all the way down the limb performing the same manipulation in sequence.

Preparation of the model

Ask the model to remove all clothing from the appropriate arm and shoulder. Shoulder straps should also be slipped off.

For a treatment in sitting

Offer the model a blanket to put over the other shoulder and wrap it obliquely across both aspects of the trunk to cross under the axilla of the arm to be massaged. The two ends can often be tucked in to secure the blanket. Check that the blanket does not hang on the floor as the model sits down. Provide a 76 cm (30″) or higher table with a top about the size of a standard pillow. Place a pillow on the table. Strap it if it is likely to slip, and cover with a cotton sheet. Place the model's arm on the pillow so that it rests in a comfortable degree of shoulder abduction and elbow flexion, and so that the pronated finger tips just reach the front of the table. (Fig. 4.1.A.)

You should stand in walk standing at the end of the table, your outer leg forward, so that you face along the forearm.

For a treatment in lying

Prepare a couch as for treatment of the lower limb, and ask the model to lie down using only two head pillows. Place a pillow along-side the trunk so that the arm can rest on it in a degree of slight abduction and flexion of the shoulder. Ensure the pronated hand is fully supported on the pillow; if not, pull the pillow down slightly leaving the shoulder area unsupported.

You should stand in walk standing just beyond the model/patient's finger tips with your outer leg forward.

To elevate the arm

Position the model in lying as for an arm treatment, but use additional pillows to ensure that each more distal joint is higher than its proximal neighbour, i.e. elbow higher than shoulder, wrist higher than elbow.

It may be necessary either to lower an adjustable couch, or for you to stand on a platform in order to reach. In the absence of either facility it is possible to work backwards, but do remember to keep looking round at the model's face.

Before starting work, uncover the whole limb in order to examine it. Follow the procedure described on p. 7, and especially check by observation the state of the skin for abrasions and dryness, and the posture of the joints which may need extra support. Then palpate—run your hand down the length of each aspect of the limb and note temperature, tenderness and muscle tone.

Effleurage

Effleurage to the whole limb

Effleurage to the upper limb is usually performed with one hand at a time while the other hand controls both the stability of the limb and

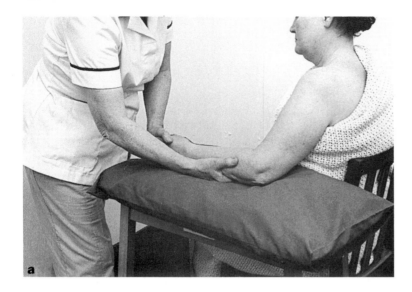

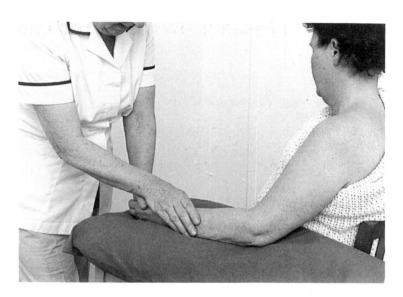

Fig. 4.2 Effleurage—third stroke with the outer hand on the forearm.

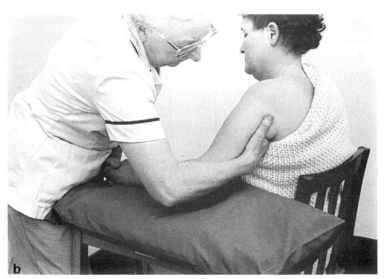

Fig. 4.1 Effleurage—first stroke with the outer hand: (a) on the ulnar aspect of the forearm, (b) at the axilla.

the position of the hand. The grasp on the hand should be with your own palm cupped so you obtain a contact with only your own palmar margins, so that a 'sticky' grasp does not arise.

Extensor aspect—grasp the pronated hand as in Fig. 4.1a with your hand nearest to the model. The working hand—the furthest from the model—is inserted under the little finger and proceeds up the ulnar border of the forearm and the medial surface of the arm, to the axilla (Fig. 4.1b). The second stroke starts on the back of the fingers, goes up the back of the forearm and the posterior surface of the arm to the axilla. Turn the forearm to mid-pronation and start the third stroke on the thumb (Fig. 4.2), continue up the radial border of the forearm and the lateral surface of the arm to the axilla.

Flexor aspect—as your working hand returns, grasp the model's hand and maintain the mid-pronation. Your former grasping hand works from the thumb (Fig. 4.3a), over the lateral border of the fore-

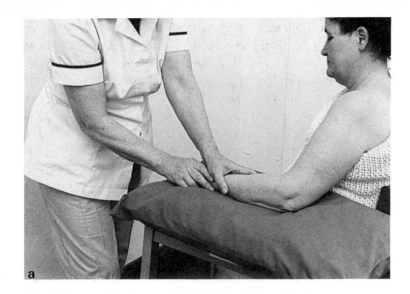

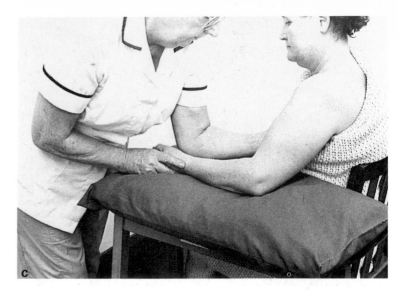

Fig. 4.3 Effleurage with the inner hand: (a) on the wrist; (b) on the arm—note the good contact; (c) at the axilla.

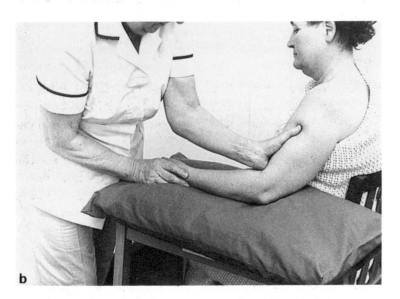

arm and the lateral surface of arm (Fig. 4.3b and c) to the axilla. Turn the palm into more supination and take the fifth stroke from the palmar aspect of the fingers over the front of the forearm and the anterior surface of the arm to the axilla. The sixth stroke goes from under the little finger, up the ulnar border of the forearm and the medial surface of the arm to the axilla.

Every stroke starts with your fingers in most contact and leading the way until you reach the model's wrist, when your working hand, now in full contact, should lie obliquely on the limb. At the axilla your hand should proceed with increased depth into the area of the space by at least the length of your working fingers and pause momentarily there.

In effect these strokes have great overlap on one another, but do create a feeling of thorough cover of the part.

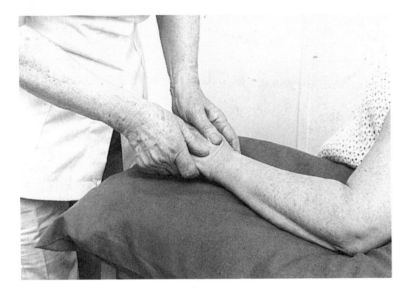

Fig. 4.4 Stroking the interosseus spaces. The same hand position is used for kneading the spaces.

Part strokes

The shoulder is effleuraged by crossing your hands to rest one each side of the shoulder. As the strokes are made, the hands are uncrossed and turned to allow the deltoid to be effleuraged as the fingers enter the axilla.

The arm may be effleuraged on its own, starting at the elbow and finishing at the axilla using the pattern of full length strokes described on pp. 33—34.

The forearm may be effleuraged either from the wrist, or the finger tips, to the anterior aspect of the elbow where some glands lie. Use the appropriate parts of the full length strokes described on pp. 33—34.

The hand may be effleuraged using the whole of your hand or individual structures may be treated by using your thumb or finger tips.

The interosseus spaces of the dorsum may be effleuraged using your thumbs in alternate spaces and working simultaneously (Fig. 4.4). The palm may be effleuraged using your thumbs or one or more fingers. By selecting anatomical features, such as abductor pollicis brevis and abductor digiti minimi to be treated simultaneously, your two thumbs can work together. The two flexors, and then the two opponens muscles can also be treated by your two thumbs, whereas three fingers will cover a less defined field.

The digits can be effleuraged in pairs—two with four, and three with five. The thumb can be effleuraged on its own. Balance the tip of each finger on your own middle phalanx and perform a stroke up one side with your index finger (Fig. 4.5a) and then up the other side with your thumb (Fig. 4.5b). This trick keeps the finger under treatment straight. If the fingers are a problem for this method, then grasp the tip gently with one of your index fingers and thumb and stroke up each side with the index finger and/or thumb of your other hand. It is more usual to stroke the sides of digits as the greatest drainage occurs there.

Kneading

All the kneading manipulations described are performed using the circling technique described on p. 11 (Fig. 2.4b). Always be aware the size of the circle must be related to the size of the area under treatment. Ensure you are working on muscle or soft tissue and avoid deep, moving pressure over bony ridges and prominences. The pressure on all the manipulations should be inwards towards the centre of the arm and with upward pressure so that you can envisage assisting venous blood and lymph flow from distal to proximal.

Double handed alternate kneading

Double handed alternate kneading of the upper limb is usually performed straight down the length of the limb, from the shoulder to

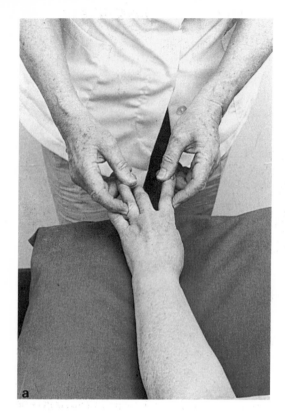

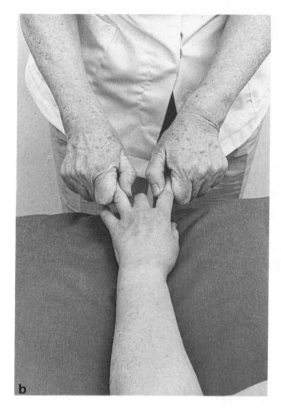

Fig. 4.5a Finger effleurage to the digits.

Fig. 4.5b Thumb effleurage to the same digits.

the finger tips, rather than sectionally as for the longer and more muscular lower limb. In consequence, the sequence of work involves careful manoeuvring of your hands so as to turn the 'corners' and to maintain full hand contact. Thus the hands start cupped over the shoulder and deltoid, encircle the upper arm to work on triceps and biceps, turn at the elbow to lie obliquely on the flexor and extensor aspects of the forearm and hand.

Start by reaching hard with your arms and your shoulder girdle so that your hands can rest over the shoulder joint, with your finger tips touching on top (Fig. 4.6a). Your elbows should be bent to allow your forearms to be parallel to the table top. Knead with alternate hand circles and inward pressure, slowly pivotting on your finger tips so that the heels of your hands move to rest over mid-line of deltoid—about six to eight circles with each hand (Fig. 4.6b).

Next, work down on deltoid in very small stages keeping your hands parallel and your thumbs touching, until your fingers can slip into the axilla. Your hands should now rest with the mid-line of each hand on the vertical mid-line of the bellies of triceps and biceps. Your fingers may overlap over the medial border of the humerus (Fig. 4.7).

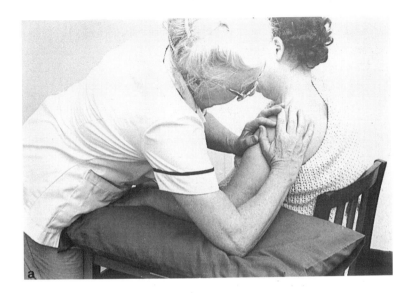

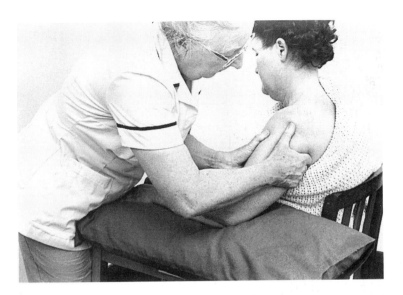

Fig. 4.7 Kneading biceps and triceps.

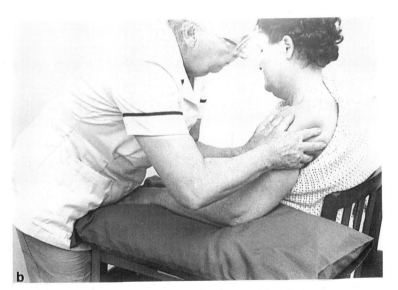

Fig. 4.6 Kneading deltoid: (a) Start. (b) Finishing positions for hands.

The kneading should now be less of a compressive manipulation, and have an element of squeeze with each hand, but, as you must keep your thumbs lying vertically and close together on each side of the lateral border of the humerus, the squeeze is effected by the thumb and thenar eminence on one side and the palm and fingers on the other side of each muscle.

Proceed down the upper arm, manoeuvring your hands gradually in the lower 1/3 so that the hand on triceps comes more to the front of the elbow, and that on biceps lies more to the back of the elbow (Fig. 4.8). Let your front hand perform stationary work, while your rear hand works and slides gradually under the medial side of the elbow and on to the flexor aspect of the forearm, followed by the other hand on to the extensor aspect of the forearm.

The kneading on the forearm is done by letting your hand on the flexors lie across the limb and in advance of your hand on the

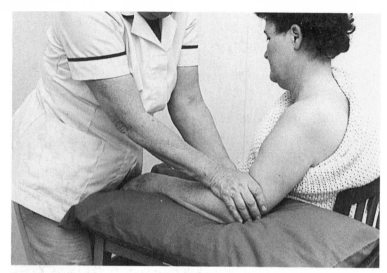

Fig. 4.8 Kneading—turning the elbow.

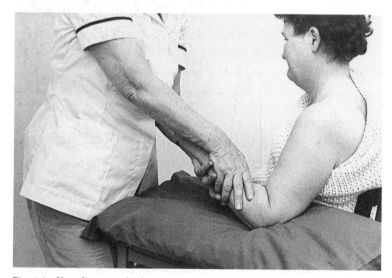

Fig. 4.9 Kneading—on the forearm—note the lifted position to facilitate the manipulation and the practitioner's hands both in contact yet in different dispositions.

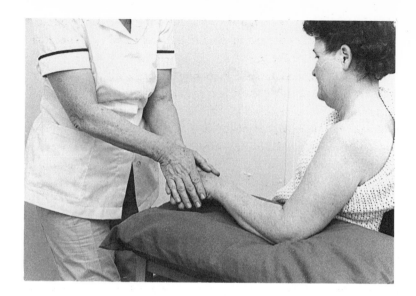

Fig. 4.10 Kneading on the hand.

extensors, which should lie obliquely, but with a more vertical alignment (Fig. 4.9). In this way, both your hands can maintain full contact, and the hand on the flexors can slightly lift the model's forearm to allow your hands to move down more easily. Your hands will catch up with each other to work at the same level on the model's palm (Fig. 4.10), continuing until his or her fingers lie in the middle of your palm. Any part of this sequence may be used to treat any specific muscle(s).

Single handed kneading

On deltoid. The whole of one of your hands may be used to knead the deltoid muscle. The outer hand is the easier to use, and your inner hand should support the model's arm just below the axilla and on the medial side, in order to give counterpressure and stabilize the area.

On triceps. Triceps is kneaded with your outer hand and counter-pressure with your other hand is given initially halfway down, then at the distal part of the biceps.

On biceps. Biceps is kneaded with your inner hand, with counter-pressure with your other hand over the mid-point and then the distal part of triceps.

On the extensors of the forearm. The forearm extensors are kneaded with your outer hand starting above the elbow flexure (remember some of the muscles take origin above the flexure), and working down to the wrist, eventually using your palm only. Support is given with your inner hand over the wrist to prevent it moving and also to raise the forearm if necessary.

The flexors of the forearm. The forearm flexors are treated in a similar way, using your inner hand starting in the elbow flexure with the whole hand, and gradually using only your palm as you work down to the wrist (Fig. 4.11). The wrist is supported with your outer hand.

The hand. The dorsum of the hand is kneaded using the palm of your outer hand, while supporting the model's palm with the palm of your inner hand. Try to cup this palm so that sticky contact of the middles of two palms is avoided. The supporting hand should be placed across the supported palm so that your fingers lie on one side, and your thumb on the other side.

Some people find it easier to learn single handed kneading before learning to use both hands.

Finger kneading

The palm of the hand is more usually kneaded with either all, or most of your fingers using flat fingers to fit over the muscle areas. Your outer hand supports the supinated hand on the dorsum to allow the middle of the palm, then the hypothenar area to be treated. Your hands change roles and the hypothenar eminence is grasped to allow your outer hand to work on the thenar area. Finger pad

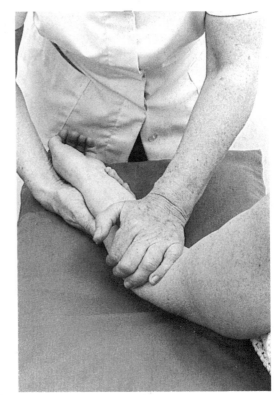

Fig. 4.11 Palmar kneading to the flexors of the forearm.

kneading can be performed on each small area and eventually on individual intrinsic muscles working from proximal to distal.

Thumb kneading

Thumb kneading is more usually performed on the flatter or smaller muscle groups of the upper limb.

The flexors and extensors of the forearm. The flexors and extensors of the forearm are treated similarly. Hold the forearm a little elevated from the pillow so that your fingers can lie on the opposite aspect. Obtain maximum contact with the length of your thumbs by keeping your forearms low and parallel with the model's forearm. Then, perform maximum size circles without skin drag, and be aware that the appearance of a wrinkle above the working thumb means that your range is enough, and skin drag will follow if you continue with pressure (Fig. 4.12). Ensure your thumbs pass one another 'off-contact' just sufficiently to allow the relaxed thumb to pass adjacent to the lateral border of the working thumb. DO NOT PRESS MOST WITH THE METACARPOPHALANGEAL JOINT of your thumb—avoid this by maintaining VERY SLIGHT flexion at this joint thus avoiding hyperextension of your thumb. The manipulation is deeper on the muscle bellies, and much lighter on the distal ½–⅓ of the forearm. The extensors are treated from above the elbow flexure anterior to the lateral epicondyle and the flexors from below the elbow flexure and distal to the medial epicondyle.

The interosseus spaces. The interosseus spaces are kneaded on the dorsal aspect using the sides of your thumbs. The manipulation has a long, narrow oval shape and is usually performed in alternate spaces i.e. 1 and 3, 2 and 4. Support the palm with your fingers, and work from proximal to distal having determined the length of the space by stroking up it (Fig. 4.4).

The thenar and hypothenar eminences are thumb kneaded by supinating the hand and:

either using both your thumbs alternately on each eminence in turn, *or* using one thumb on each eminence and selecting the appropriate pairs of small muscles. The abductor digiti minimi and abductor

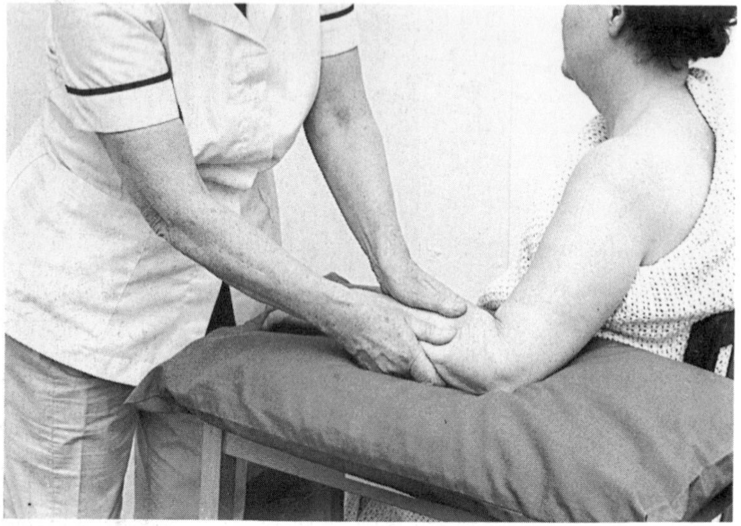

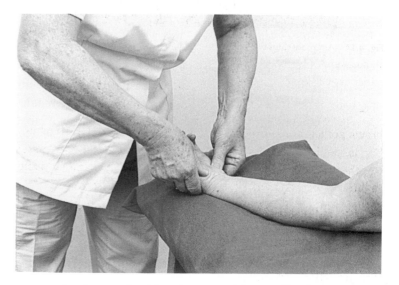

Fig. 4.12 Thumb kneading to the extensors of the forearm. Note the skin wrinkle at the tip of the right thumb.

Fig. 4.13 Simultaneous thumb kneading to the abductor pollicis brevis and abductor digiti minimi.

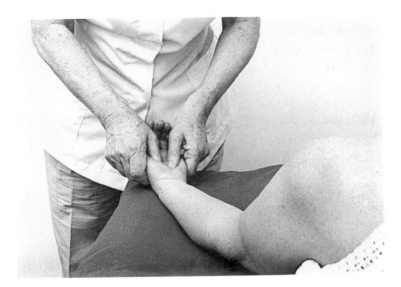

Fig. 4.14 Alternate thumb kneading to the centre of the palm.

or hold the proximal phalanx of two alternate fingers cupped on the middle phalanx of your index finger. Your thumb pad should be on the dorsum of the same area of the same finger. Now, squeeze knead by working first with your thumb then with your cupped finger while counterpressing with the opposite component, and proceed from proximal to distal working with both your hands simultaneously (Fig. 4.16). The other two fingers are treated in the same way, then the thumb is treated alone, using one hand while your other hand stabilizes the model's hand.

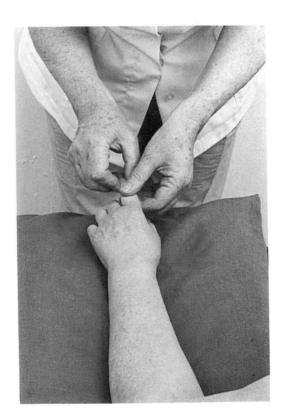

Fig. 4.15 Kneading one digit at once.

brevis pollicis are kneaded simultaneously and together, the flexor brevis pollicis (Fig. 4.13) and flexor digiti minimi are treated together and simultaneously, then the centre of the palm (adductor pollicis) is kneaded with both thumbs alternately (Fig. 4.14). This sequence prevents the wrist from being rocked sideways as the manipulations are performed. Use your thumb pads or tips for these manipulations.

The fingers. The fingers can be kneaded in two ways. Turn the hand into pronation and:

either hold the tip of one finger in one hand, and use the thumb pad and pad of the index finger of the other hand, one on the front and one on the back of the finger near the cleft to knead both aspects at once or first one aspect, then the other (Fig. 4.15),

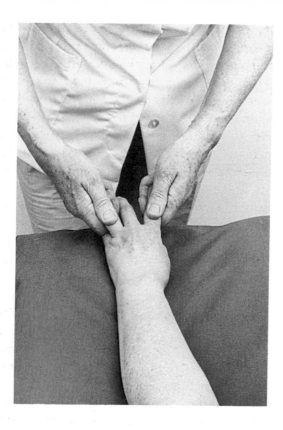

Fig. 4.16 Kneading
two digits at once.

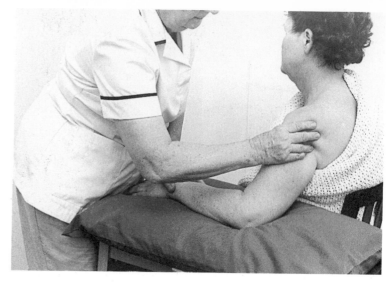

Fig. 4.17 Picking up to deltoid—note the 'C' shape of the hand.

Picking up

Picking up on the upper limb muscles is usually performed with one hand at once, and from proximal to distal. The operator's outer hand works on deltoid, triceps and brachioradialis and the inner hand on the biceps brachii and the forearm flexors. The free hand stabilizes the limb adjacent to the working hand. Progress should be in small stages of about 1—2 cm (½"—¾") at a time.

Deltoid is picked up using your outer hand with your inner hand stabilizing on the medial side of the arm near the elbow. Use a 'C' for-

mation of the hand (see Fig 2.14) and find the bony margins of the spine of the scapula, the acromion process and anterior border of the clavicle. Now slip down on to the deltoid and *totally off* the bone. Keep your palm in contact with deltoid all the time so that you compress the whole muscle but pick up rather less of it. Your forearm should be parallel with the model's forearm and remain so as you work. The 'pick up' is performed by extending your wrist after you have grasped the muscle and you should neither pivot on your thumb and finger tips, nor lever on the heel of your hand (Fig. 4.17). A vulnerable bony area is the lateral border of the bicipital groove and your thumb should always lie lateral to it and not on it. As the muscle narrows, you narrow the 'C' shape of your hand to almost a 'V' shape.

Triceps is treated by sliding your hand from the tendon of deltoid to the back of the arm near the axilla, so that you encompass the triceps

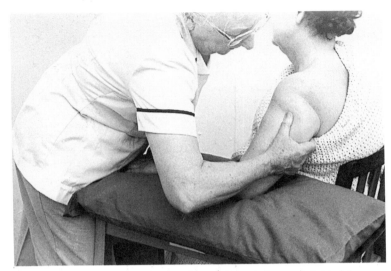

Fig. 4.18 Picking up to triceps—note the practitioner's forearm is behind the model's arm and the hand is 'C' shaped.

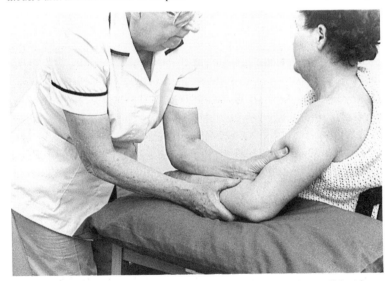

Fig. 4.19 Picking up to biceps—note the practitioner's forearm is parallel with that of the model.

muscle belly (Fig. 4.18). Your finger tips should lie posterior to the medial border of the humerus, and the length of your thumb should be posterior to the lateral border of the humerus. Again, keep the whole of your palm in contact with the muscle belly, and your forearm low and parallel with that of the model. Your stabilizing hand should be on the biceps near the elbow.

Biceps—as triceps is completed, your other (stabilizing) hand slides out of the way and up to the proximal part of biceps. Again, your finger tips and length of your thumb lie in front of the adjacent bony borders of the humerus with your palm in full contact, and your forearm parallel with the model's forearm (Fig. 4.19). As you work down the biceps muscle, your other hand should initially stabilize on the back of the elbow and move out of the way to the outside of the wrist which is lifted and the palm supinated, so that the working hand can continue to the tendon of insertion of biceps then slip medially to the:

Forearm flexors. These muscles are picked up using the 'V' formation of the hand (Fig. 2.15) with your fingers on the posteromedial aspect, and your thumb on the anterolateral aspect. Again, maintain full palmar contact and narrow the 'V' as you proceed down the forearm to the wrist.

Brachioradialis requires the use of your outer hand, so effect a smooth change by grasping and supporting at the wrist with the previously working hand, and sliding your outer hand up the length of brachioradialis to just above the elbow flexure (Fig. 4.20). Keep the forearm lifted to relax the muscle, and pick up using a 'V' formation until you reach the musculotendinous junction, which is two thirds of the way down the forearm. Many people continue to perform a picking up action as a squeeze on both aspects of the distal end of the forearm to preserve continuity of contact. At this point in a sequence on the arm, the forearm extensors are often thumb kneaded. Alternatively, you can return to the shoulder area to perform wringing.

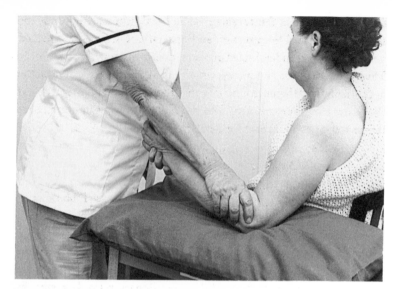

Fig. 4.20 Picking up to brachioradialis—note the 'V' shape of the hand.

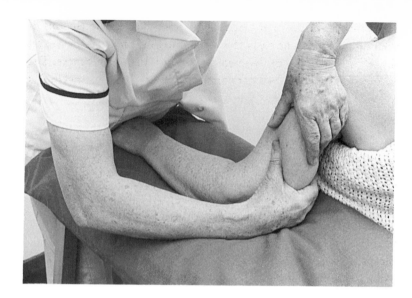

Fig. 4.21 Wringing to the triceps—note the practitioner's long reach to avoid dragging with her fingers.

Wringing

Wringing is most easily performed on the long muscles of triceps and biceps brachii. It is possible to wring a flabby or very relaxed deltoid, but the muscle is so short that it presents difficulties in performance. **Deltoid and triceps** can be wrung by pivoting your stance and body so that you are nearer to the model and your nearest foot is between the model and the table. In both cases, your fingers should be on the back of the arm and your thumbs on the front and medial side. Ensure that these components of your hands are not lying over the adjacent bony border—the bicipital groove in the case of deltoid, and the lateral border of the humerus in the case of the triceps (Fig. 4.21). The muscles should be grasped at their most proximal end and you should work to the distal end and, perhaps return. Try to proceed in small stages so that your hands move about 2–4 cm (1″–1½″) at a time and move constantly.

Biceps. For biceps, you will need to move your stance slightly to the outer side of the arm support and, again, use your fingers on the medial side anterior to the medial border of the humerus, and your thumbs on the lateral side anterior to the lateral border of the humerus. Again work from most proximal to the distal part of the muscle and perhaps return and in similar small stages as on the triceps.

Be very careful in wringing these muscles not to drag on the skin and to keep your hand changes of direction very smooth. Dry hands are a great help in ensuring smooth, non-dragging work.

Brachioradialis. The belly of brachioradialis may be wrung using your thumb pads and the pads of your index, middle and sometimes ring fingers. The model's forearm should be fully supported in mid-pronation and supination.

Hand muscles. Tiny wringing manipulations done with the tips of your index fingers and sides of your thumb tips can be performed on the intrinsic muscles of the thenar and hypothenar eminences. The two abductor and two flexor muscles are more easily treated in this way.

Muscle shaking

Deltoid. The shorter deltoid muscle can be shaken using your outer hand. Take care not to bounce on the bicipital groove with your thumb.

Triceps is shaken, again, using your outer hand and proceeding from near the axilla to the elbow (Fig. 4.22).

Biceps is shaken using your inner hand, proceeding from near the axilla to the musculotendinous junction.

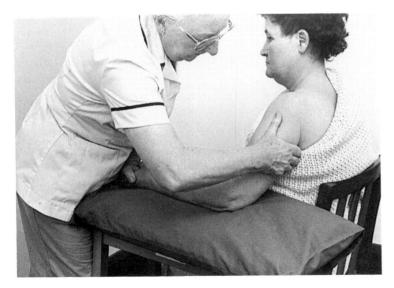

Fig. 4.22 Muscle shaking—note the loose grasp.

Brachioradialis. In the forearm, a bulky brachioradialis may be shaken using the thumb pad and the lateral side of the flexed phalanges of the index finger of your inner or outer hands.

The hand. In the hand, you may be able to shake the bulk of both the hypothenar and thenar eminences and, in some subjects to select and shake the abductor brevis pollicis and abductor digiti minimi using the tips of your thumb and index finger.

Muscle rolling

Muscle rolling can be performed on each of the upper limb muscles which can be picked up, and this manipulation is often easier to perform on brachioradialis than either wringing or picking up.

Place your thumbs and fingers as though you intended to do wringing—as described above, and push the muscle belly gently first with both of your thumbs while your fingers relax but stay in contact, then pull with the distal phalanges of all your fingers while your thumbs relax but stay in contact. Proceed along the length of each muscle working down, then up, with this rocking action. Work fairly quickly and with a slight pressure inward towards mid line of the limb so that the muscle rolls from side to side.

Muscle rolling can also be performed with the thumb and finger tips on the two flexor and two abductor muscles of the thenar and hypothenar eminences. This manipulation can also be used to roll or 'rock' scars and adherent tissue.

Hacking and clapping

Hacking and clapping are usually performed successively to first one aspect of the upper limb, then to the other, so that the limb is moved only once.

With the model's forearm pronated, start at the posterior axilla and work down the posterior part of deltoid, triceps (reach round to

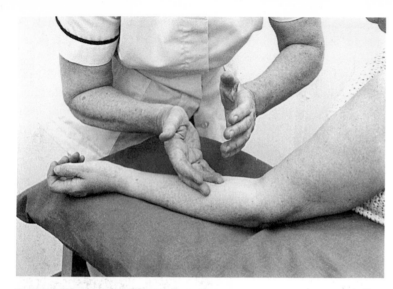

Fig. 4.23 Hacking to the forearm flexors.

the back of the arm to do so) and then on to the forearm extensors. You may need to stop the hacking at mid forearm in bony subjects, but should be able to clap on to the dorsum of the hand. Stand nearer the model for this work.

Turn the forearm to supination and lift the elbow medially, so that the limb rests comfortably on the support. Either stand on the outer side of the support, or step nearer to the model's feet, and starting at the axilla work down the front of deltoid, biceps, the forearm flexors (Fig. 4.23) and the palm of the hand, and reverse up the limb.

By working in this way you will strike the muscle fibres across their longitudinal axis.

In both lines of work you should:

1 work in a zig zag fashion on each muscle if it is bulky or wide enough,

2 avoid bony prominences and large tendons and jump over them:

- at the back,   the radial groove
  the lateral epicondyle
  the posterior surface of the distal part of the radius and ulna
- at the front,   the tendon of deltoid
  the bicipital groove
  the tendon of biceps
  the medial epicondyle
  the prominent carpal bones.

Clapping is performed in a similar pattern using a more cupped hand on the more slender parts of the limb (Fig. 4.24).

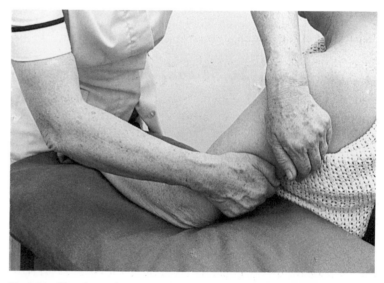

Fig. 4.24 Clapping to the upper arm.

Chapter 5: Massage to the Lower Limb

Preparation of the model

Ask the model to remove all clothing below the waist except briefs or pants. If the model has no suitable underwear, provide him or her with either disposable pants or a loin cloth. Check that the feet are clean and not malodorous. If necessary, ask the model/patient to wash (use the excuse that a foot soak will help the treatment).

Preparation of the treatment couch

Cover the couch with an underblanket and cotton sheet, and fix them in position with straps. Provide two pillows for the model's head, and either one large pillow to go under both knees, or two small pillows to go one under each knee.

Treatment of the lower limb with the model supine

If possible the model should lie flat, but some people prefer or some patients may need, to have the elevating, head end of the couch raised so that half lying is the position used. Avoid an angle of elevation of the backrest of more than 45° so that drainage is not impeded. Cover the legs with a cotton sheet and blanket and provide a second small blanket for the upper part of the body. If the lower limb needs elevation for the treatment of oedema, then it should be supported by pillows or by the raising of the end of the couch at no more than 45° of elevation (Fig. 5.1). In this case, the trunk must not be raised 45° as well. Provide additional head pillows instead of elevating the head end of the couch.

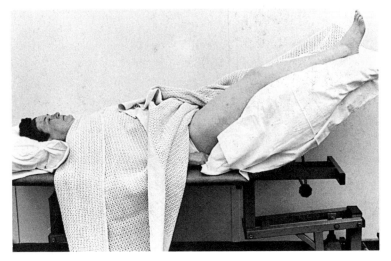

Fig. 5.1 The lower limb elevated.

When working on an elevated lower limb, it may be necessary either to lower an adjustable couch or, if the couch is of fixed height, for you to stand on a low platform in order to reach. In the absence of either of these facilities, it is possible to turn round and face the model's feet and work backwards, but do remember to keep looking round at the model's face (Fig. 5.2).

Treatment of the lower limb with the model prone

(To gain access to the posterior aspect of the lower limb.)

The model lies prone, with head and abdomen supported as for

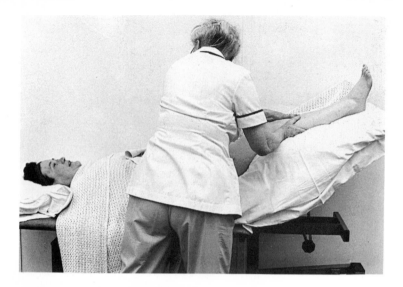

Fig. 5.2 The lower limb treated by working backwards. Note the practitioner is observing the model's face.

back massage (p. 66). Place one pillow under both ankles to allow a little flexion at both knees, and sufficient pillows under the calf of the limb to be treated so that the knee is flexed no more than 45° (Fig. 8.8). Ensure that the ankle is supported in some plantarflexion. This position is suitable for treatment of the hamstrings and/or the calf. If insufficient pillows are available, the model's ankle can rest on your shoulder, but arrange yourself carefully so that if possible you can half sit (perch) on the edge of the couch as the calf can feel very heavy by the end of the treatment and more so if you stand to work and support the limb.

Before starting work always uncover the whole limb in order to examine it. Follow the procedure described on p. 7 and especially check by observation:

• the state of the skin for dryness, callosities, and abrasions, the pre-

sence of any varicose vessels, the posture of the joints which may need extra supports.

Then palpate—run your hand down the length of each aspect of the limb and note:

• temperature, tenderness and muscle tone.

Treatment of the whole lower limb with the model supine

Effleurage

Effleurage to the whole limb

Stand with your rear foot distal to the model's foot, and your forward foot level with the model's calf. Both hands usually work together; your nearside hand on the sole of the foot and more medial aspect of the limb, and your more lateral hand on the dorsum of the foot and the more lateral aspect of the limb.

There are two methods of working on the foot:

1 Each hand starts with the fingers over the toes (Fig. 5.3a), that on the dorsum, traverses to the anterolateral side of the ankle slightly in front of that on the plantar aspect, which passes under the instep to the anteromedial side of the ankle.

2 The alternative method of working on the foot is only different for the hand on the dorsum. For each stroke, this hand starts with the whole hand on the dorsum of the foot, the fingers over the toes and palm over the tarsus. The heel of this hand is near to the lateral malleolus. The stroke with this hand is initiated by pivoting it with some depth on the dorsum of the foot, so that your fingers turn to lie on the outer side of the foot and then proceed as described above (Fig. 5.3b). This method is useful where there is a painful ankle joint or foot as the counterpressures of the hands prevent unwanted ankle plantarflexion which can be inadvertently caused by Method 1.

Whichever method you have used you must now abduct and

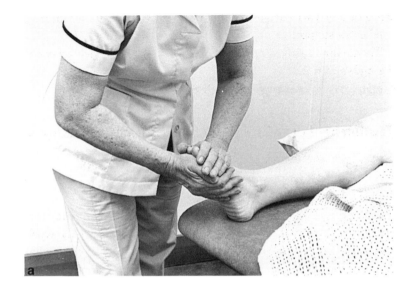

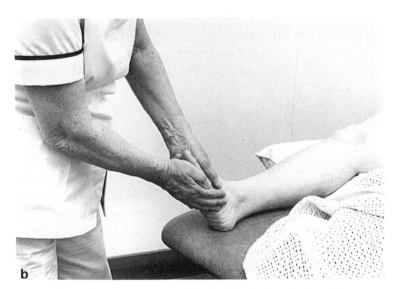

Fig. 5.3 Optional starting positions of (a, b) of the hands on the foot, for effleurage to the lower limb.

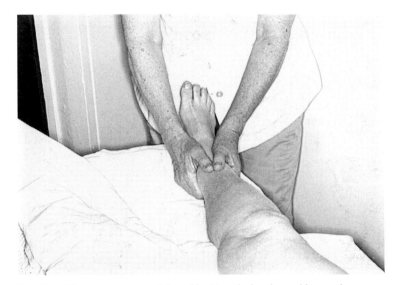

Fig. 5.4 Effleurage continues at the ankle. Note the hands moulding to the part.

extend your thumbs so that your hands span first the sides (Fig. 5.4), then the front of the ankle and proceed up the front of the leg (Fig. 5.5) over the knee and thigh to the femoral triangle where you should increase your pressure and pause briefly. Throughout this part of the stroke, your hands fit together (Fig. 5.6) with the thumb of your outer hand lying alongside the index finger of your inner hand. For each successive stroke, your hands should fit together in this way as they come round to the front of the thigh and continue to the femoral triangle, where overpressure is given with a slight pause. The next stroke starts in the same way, but your fingers pass behind the malleoli so that your hands can continue up the medial and lateral aspects of the limb (Fig. 5.7). Your outer hand should, again, be slightly in advance of your medial hand and both move more anteriorly at the junction of the upper and middle ⅓ of the thigh so that they encompass the femoral triangle. The third stroke starts like

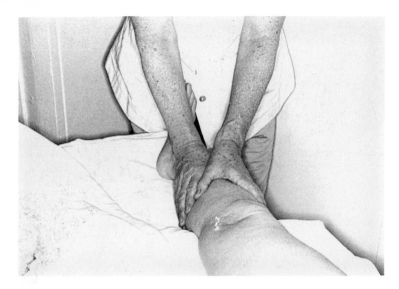

Fig. 5.5   Stroke 1—effleurage to the front of the calf.

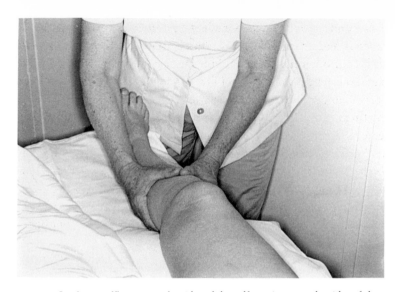

Fig. 5.7   Stroke 2—effleurage to the sides of the calf continues up the sides of the thigh.

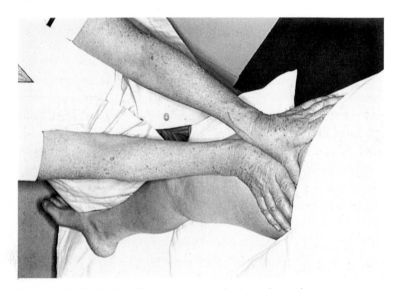

Fig. 5.6   The finish of an effleurage stroke at the femoral triangle.

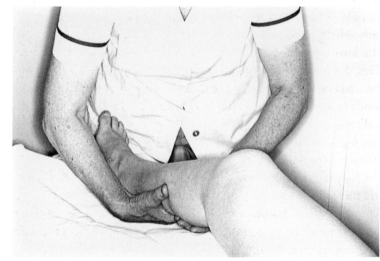

Fig. 5.8   Stroke 3—effleurage to the back of the calf continues up the back of the thigh.

the second stroke, but at the malleoli your fingers pass the tendocalcaneous and proceed up the posterior aspect of the limb (Fig. 5.8) with your outer hand slightly in front of your inner hand. You will have to extend *your back* and lift *the model's limb* very slightly to proceed under the thigh from the back of the knee. At the upper ⅓ of the thigh, your hands circumnavigate to the front to finish at the femoral triangle. Pressure has to be varied to allow for the smaller ankle, bulky muscular calf, more bony knee and bulky muscular thigh. This can be best controlled by adjusting your foot positions and ensuring your arms start to 'reach' before your body moves. You should feel your shoulder girdle protracting to assist the reaching process. At no time should you bend either your hips or your back.

Part strokes of effleurage

The thigh can be effleuraged alone if the patterns of strokes previously described start at the knee and proceed to the femoral triangle. The posterior stroke is started by sliding the hands from each side to underneath the knee.

The knee is effleuraged by crossing your hands above the patella (Figs. 5.9 a and b), drawing them backwards on each side of it until the heels of your hands meet below the patella, then turning your hands to allow your fingers to pass behind the knee over the popliteal fossa.

The leg is effleuraged from foot or ankle to the popliteal fossa, following the lines of work for the whole lower limb.

The foot is effleuraged by starting in one of the two described ways and finishing at the ankle.

The interosseus spaces are effleuraged using the sides of your thumbs, meantime supporting the plantar aspect of the foot with your fingers (Fig. 5.10).

The toes. The big toe is dealt with on its own. The tip is supported on the tip of your middle finger, and your thumb and index finger

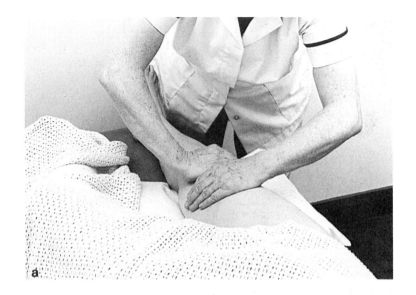

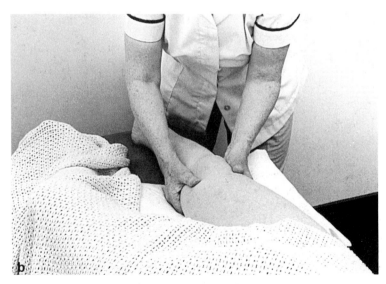

Fig. 5.9 Effleurage to the knee: (a) start, (b) finish.

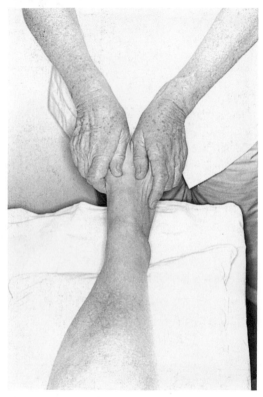

Fig. 5.10 The position of the hands for either an effleurage stroke or kneading to the interosseus spaces of the foot.

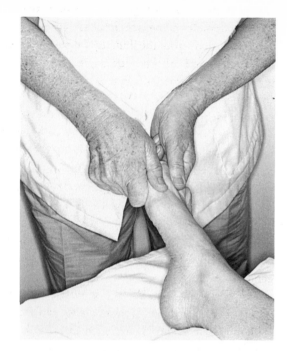

Fig. 5.11 The position of the hands for either an effleurage stroke or kneading to the toes.

stroke one up each side (Fig. 5.11). As the lateral four toes are so small, you may find you have to stroke the sides of each toe separately, balancing the tip of each toe on your middle finger and stroking up the toe on one side with your thumb and then on the other side with your index finger.

Take care:

• to follow the basic rules for effleurage, especially ensuring you do not give maximum pressure with the leading edge of your hands;

To continue working on the thigh, cover the leg and foot with part of the blanket.

Kneading

All the kneading manipulations on the lower limb are performed using the circling technique described on p. 11 (Fig. 2.4b) with modifications for the size of the area under treatment. Ensure you are working on muscle or soft tissue and avoid deep, moving pressure over bony ridges and prominences. The pressure of all the manipulations should be inwards to the centre of the limb with an upward inclination so that you can envisage assisting venous blood and lymph flow from distal to proximal.

Kneading to the thigh

The thigh is usually treated with double handed, alternate kneading dealing with the medial and lateral aspects together, and the anterior and posterior aspects together. Consider the anatomy—the hamstrings extend from the ischial tuberosity to the tibia, and the rectus femoris extends from the ilium to the patella. Two groups extending the whole length of the thigh so, except on the medial aspect, the manipulations start as high as your hands can be placed and continue to the knee.

The adductor group occupies most of the upper medial half of the thigh, and vastus medialis the lower half. On the lateral side, is vastus lateralis, covered by the strong fascia lata and extending most of the length of that side. Thus, there is a long length on the lateral side, and less than half that length on the medial aspect. The adductors are rarely treated in a routine practice. Specific manipulations may be used in groin strains of adductor longus tendon, but on the whole, the upper medial aspect of the thigh is not massaged as the cutaneous nerve supply of the area is shared by the external genitalia.

Stand in walk standing at the level of the lower calf with your outer foot forward. For the lateral and medial lines of work, the lateral hand initiates the kneading at half tempo and works down the thigh until it is opposite the medial hand, which is resting ready on the middle of the medial aspect. This hand now works alternately with the other hand to continue to the knee (Fig. 5.12a). For the anterior and posterior lines of work, the anterior and posterior muscles are kneaded *either* by remaining in the same posture as for the lateral/medial aspects and inserting your nearer (medial) hand under the thigh from the inside to work on the hamstrings, while your outer hand works on the anterior aspect (Fig. 5.12b), *or* by turning your body more to face across the thigh, you then insert your hand nearest to the model's hip (outer hand) under the thigh from the outside and the further, formerly medial hand works on the anterior aspect (Fig. 5.12c).

In order to work deeply on these great muscle masses you must lean forward with a straight back, working always with your hands

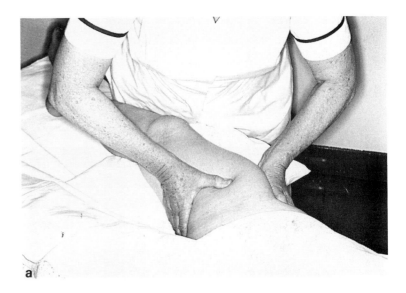

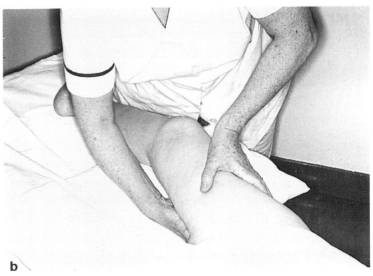

Fig. 5.12 Kneading—the thigh: (a) medial and lateral aspects, (b) one method for the anterior and posterior aspects, (c) overleaf.

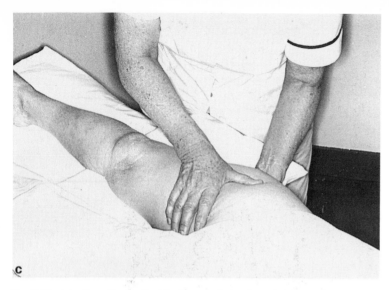

Fig. 5.12 (c) alternative method for the anterior or posterior aspects.

in front of the level of your shoulders. As your hands proceed down the thigh, transfer your weight from your forward to your rear foot, but your weight must also be transferred constantly from one foot to the other by pivoting your pelvis. Your weight should be more on the forward foot when kneading with the outer hand, and more on the rear foot when kneading with the inner hand.

When you work on the thigh muscles keep the anatomy constantly in mind and envisage straight lines down the length of the *centres* of the muscles you are working upon. Keep the middle of your hand along this line so that you do not work across two muscles or muscle groups at once, which is much harder work for you as well as less effective and less comfortable for the model.

Kneading round the knee

Whole-handed kneading round the knee should extend from just above the superior margin of the synovial membrane to a hand width below the flexure of the knee so that you encompass all the structures in the region.

Start with both hands on the anterior aspect with the heels of the hands touching above the patella. Work down, letting the heels of your hands divide round the patella to avoid working over it. Let the heels of your hands meet again below the patella. Next, insert each hand from opposite sides under the lower thigh until your fingers overlap. Now work down on this aspect, covering the same level as in the previous line of work.

Thumb kneading round the patella

Use the maximum length of your thumbs and work:
either with your thumbs one on each side of the patella—i.e. starting near each other and dividing round the bone margin (Fig. 5.13a),
or with both thumbs working adjacent and alternately round every aspect of the patella margin (Fig. 5.13b).

Finger kneading at the knee

Use your finger tips to work on each side of the bony areas of the knee with your thumbs resting on an adjacent area. Place your finger tips in a linear formation on first one side, then the other, of the tendons of the hamstrings at the knee so that one hand is on biceps femoris and the other on the semimembranosus and semitendonosus tendons.

If you are practising the kneading manipulations to increase your skill, continue on to the leg and foot—in which case, cover the thigh with the blanket and uncover the leg and foot and continue as described below. If you are working on each area to give treatment, then complete all the manipulations for the thigh, in which case turn

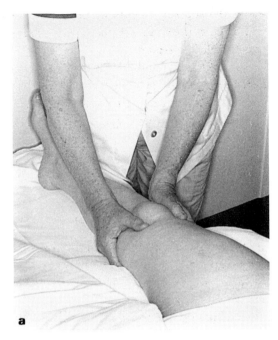

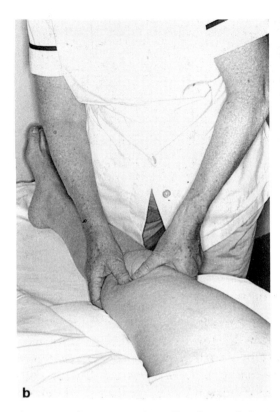

Fig. 5.13 Optional methods (a, b) of thumb kneading to the knee.

to pp. 59—63 for the petrissage manipulations, and to pp. 63—65 for the tapôtement manipulations for the thigh.

Kneading the calf muscles

Stand in walk standing distal to the model's feet. The lower limb may be flexed with the foot resting flat on the couch to give better access, but it is feasible to perform the double handed kneading with the limb flat, though you should push the knee pillow higher under the thigh so that the lower edge is at the level of the knee flexure. Insert one of your hands from each side under the calf so

that your fingers overlap. On the medial side, the heel of your hand must be behind the medial border of the tibia, and the heel of your hand on the lateral side must be behind the line of the fibula (Fig. 5.14).

As you knead, ensure your fingers stay overlapped. Some people actually interlock their fingers, but you may find this difficult as you work down to the narrower ankle area. Your hands should overlap more as the manipulation proceeds down the limb so that eventually one is superimposed on the other. The deeper hand performs the kneading, and the outer hand circles with it and reinforces if need be.

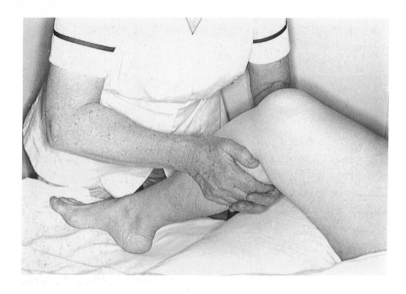

Fig. 5.14 Kneading to the calf muscles. The knee has been flexed for the photograph.

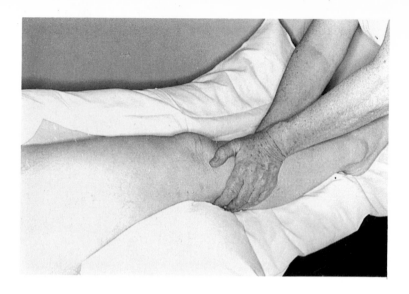

Fig. 5.15 Palmar kneading to the anterior tibial muscles.

Palmar kneading to the anterior tibial muscles

Place your palm, thumb closed to it, over the upper extremities of the anterior tibial group with your fingers off-contact. Stabilize the limb with your other hand. Work down the muscle, coming more to the front of the limb as the muscle bulk diminishes, and continue on to the dorsum of the foot to the insertions of the muscles on the medial aspect of the foot, and on the toes (Fig. 5.15).

Palmar kneading on the peronei

Place the palm of your hand, thumb closed to it and fingers off-contact, on the upper limit of the peronei and work down the lateral aspect of the calf to above the lateral malleolus.

Kneading to the foot

Move the pillow to support the leg and to keep the model's heel off the couch. Place your outer hand on the dorsum of the foot, with your fingers lying laterally and your thumb below the medial malleolus (Fig. 5.16). Place your other hand on the sole of the foot, with your thenar eminence fitted into the medial longitudinal arch, fingers on the lateral side and thumb under the medial malleolus.

Work down the foot with a kneading manipulation which should also squeeze. You will find that you must always maintain some pressure with both hands all the time, or the foot will rock back and forth. Continue kneading until the toe tips rest in the middle of your palms.

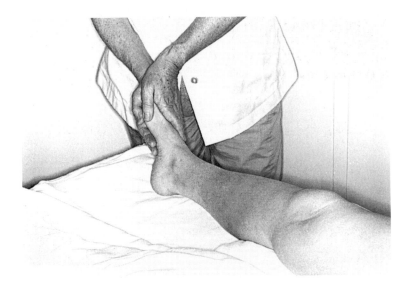

Fig. 5.16 Kneading to the foot.

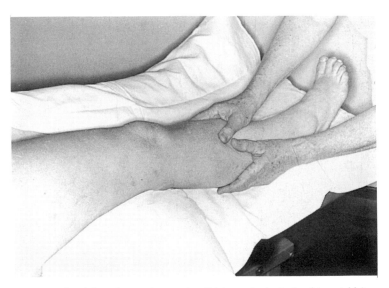

Fig. 5.17 Thumb kneading to the anterior tibial muscles (note the skin wrinkle).

Thumb kneading to the anterior tibial muscles

Medially rotate the whole limb slightly, and place both thumbs as flat as possible on the upper extremity of the bulk of the anterior tibial muscles. The remainder of your hands should rest round the calf, so that the palms are off-contact, but the fingers are supporting the limb (Fig. 5.17). Carry out a kneading manipulation so that the thumbs work throughout their length and, by bypassing one another, the whole width of the muscle group is treated. As you work down the part, move your line of work anteriorly so that your thumbs finish on the front of the ankle and can proceed if desired over the tendons to their distal attachments on the tarsus and phalanges.

Thumb kneading the peroneal muscles

Medially rotate the whole limb and bend yourself a little sideways, so that you can place both thumb pads on the upper extremity of the peronei (Fig. 5.18). The remainder of your hands rest round the calf as described above. Using only the thumb pads, work down the length of the muscles and on to the tendons as they lie behind the lateral malleolus.

Thumb kneading the dorsum of the foot

Palpate the muscle belly of the extensor digitorum brevis just anterior to the lateral malleolus. Place both thumb pads over the muscle belly and, with your fingers firmly supporting the sole

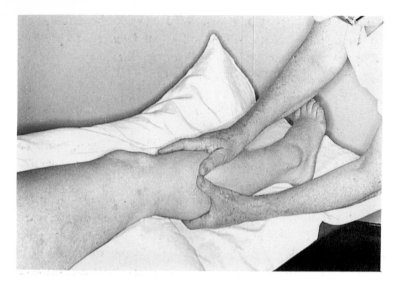

Fig. 5.18 Thumb kneading to the peroneal muscles.

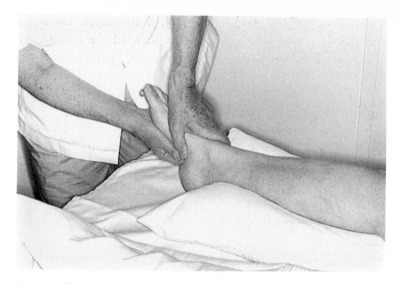

Fig. 5.19 Thumb kneading to abductor hallucis.

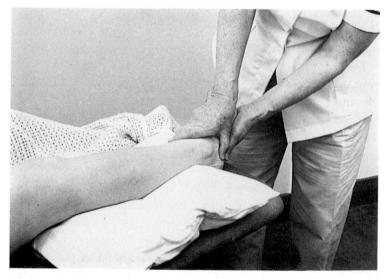

Fig. 5.20 Thumb kneading to abductor digiti minimi (note the practitioner's body is turned and sideflexed to obtain even access).

of the foot, work along the dorsum using an increasing amount of the length of your thumbs until you are working over the dorsum of the four medial toes.

Thumb kneading to the sole of the foot

Lean over to put your thumbs over the medial aspect of the foot, to treat abductor hallucis and the plantar aspect in mid-line (Fig. 5.19). Turn, as in Fig. 5.20, to put your thumbs over the lateral aspect of the foot, to treat abductor digiti minimi. Palpate the line of abductor hallucis muscle belly and, using your thumb pads, work from the heel to the base of the big toe with your finger tips resting on the outer side of the foot (Fig. 5.19).

Next, lean further over, and work under the middle of the plantar aspect from the heel to the transverse arch.

Turn your body to the position in Fig. 5.20, palpate the line of abductor digiti minimi and, using your thumb pads, knead along the muscle to the little toe. Avoid tickling by using considerable depth.

Thumb kneading to the interosseus spaces

Palpate two alternate spaces, either *one* and *three* or *two* and *four*, and place the sides of your thumb pads in two spaces at the proximal end. Work simultaneously with both thumbs with a narrow oval manoeuvre along the length of the space. Your fingers should be giving counterpressure on the plantar aspect of the foot (Fig. 5.10). Repeat for the other two spaces.

Thumb and finger kneading to the toes

The big toe is kneaded by using your medial hand, with your thumb on the dorsum and your index finger curved round the medial, plantar and lateral aspects of the big toe. The manipulation is a squeeze knead performed from proximal to distal (Fig. 5.11).

The four small toes are kneaded by holding each of them between your thumb tip and the tip of your index finger, and working along the length of the dorsal and plantar aspects (Fig. 5.11). You may need to hold each toe by its tip and work on that one toe alone, or to work on two alternate toes at once, depending on their state of flexion and rigidity.

Picking up

Picking up on the thigh

Picking up may be performed on the vastus medialis, rectus femoris and vastus intermedius, and on vastus lateralis with the model supine. The hamstrings can be most easily treated with the model prone, but from the supine position, access may be obtained by flexing the knee a little and rolling the thigh laterally. To perform picking up on these muscles individually, single-handed work described on pp. 15–17 is practised first.

SINGLE-HANDED PICKING UP, TO DOUBLE-HANDED, ALTERNATE PICKING UP

It is wiser initially to practise on an accessible muscle group, and the anterior muscles are those of choice. Stand in walk standing opposite the thigh and facing the couch.

Place your hand which is nearer the model's foot on the proximal end of rectus femoris, and practise the technique described on pp. 15–17, working until your hand reaches the patella. Keep your other hand in contact with the upper thigh. Change hands, and work with the hand nearer the model's head from just above the patella to the groin. Each hand thus travels backwards.

When you have practised enough to control your hand and body movements, then start to work forwards with each hand. This

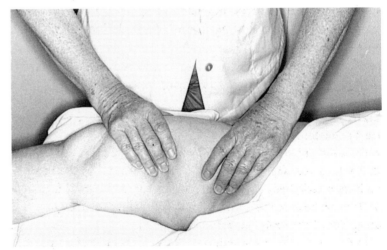

Fig. 5.21 Picking up—double-handed alternate—to the anterior thigh muscles.

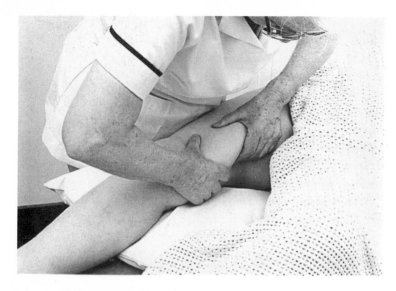

Fig. 5.22 Picking up—double-handed alternate—to the vastus medialis (note the practitioner leans forwards to keep the forearms parallel with the limb).

means that on the RELEASE your hand slides forward, instead of backwards before re-imposing pressure on the part.

Skill in working in either direction can then be combined to working backwards with one hand, and forwards with the other, thus passing the lifted tissues from hand to hand (Fig. 5.21).

The same procedure should then be practised on the vastus medialis, but in order to do so, you must lean forward with a straight back, so that your shoulders are parallel with and over the medial side of the thigh (Fig. 5.22). Start the line of work either at mid-thigh, or at the level of the knee flexure. For the lateral aspect of the thigh, you will have to take a half pace back with your rear foot, and bend both knees and hips to allow your forearms to be level with the outer side of the thigh. Start the line of work at the level of the knee flexure, or just below the great trochanter of the femur. Heavier 'ON' pressure will be necessary to gain any effect through the tough, late-

ral fascial structures, and in some cases no movement may be possible. For treatment, give extra kneading to this area.

Access to the hamstrings is effected by flexing the model's knee and lifting the thigh into lateral rotation. By using flexion at your hips and some flexion of your upper back, you can reach round the medial side of the thigh and work on the hamstrings from either the knee flexure, or proximally as high as it is possible to reach under the thigh.

DOUBLE HANDED, SIMULTANEOUS PICKING UP

Double handed, simultaneous picking up may also be performed on the anterior quadriceps (see p. 17 and Fig. 2.16).

If the model lies prone, with one or two pillows under the calf to flex the knee a little, as described on pp. 47–48 the hamstrings can also be picked up as described for the vastus intermedius and rectus femoris. If the muscle bellies are very bulky, use two lines of work, one for biceps femoris and one for semimembranosus and semitendonosus. The extent of work is from just below the ischial tuberosity to the knee flexure.

Picking up on the calf

The calf muscles can also be picked up with the model either supine or in prone lying. Only the muscle bulk can be picked up, but the tendocalcaneous is usually wrung.

Stand in walk standing level with the calf. With the model supine the best access is gained by rolling the whole lower limb laterally, and working from the knee flexure to the musculotendinous junction (Fig. 5.23). If the muscle is very bulky, it is sometimes possible to work from the lateral aspect as well, in which case the lower limb should be rolled medially.

With the model in prone lying, and the foot and calf supported on one or two pillows, the calf muscles will be relaxed at the knee and

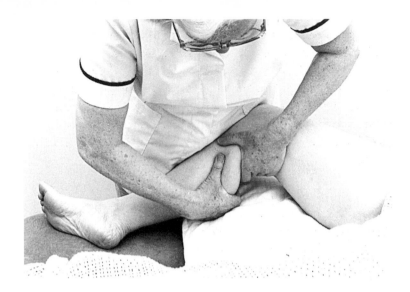

Fig. 5.23 Picking up—double handed alternate—to the calf muscles.

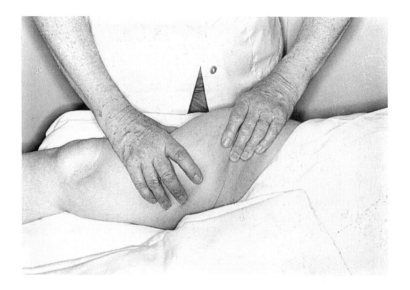

Fig. 5.24 Wringing—to the anterior thigh muscles.

ankle, and the upper ⅔ of the calf can be picked up from the knee flexure to the musculotendinous junction.

Wringing

Wringing on the thigh

Each of the thigh muscles can be treated by wringing. Your starting position, the lines of work and length of muscle treated are the same as for picking up, with the greatest effects being achieved on the anterior, medial and posterior muscle groups, in that order (Fig. 5.24). The manipulation can be difficult on the lateral aspect. Do ensure that you have lifted the muscle and are not just wringing the skin and subcutaneous tissues. The model may be supine or in prone lying for wringing the hamstrings.

Wringing on the calf

In exactly the same way as for the thigh, the calf can be treated by wringing. With the model supine, the medial half of the calf can easily be lifted and have wringing performed on it; the lateral side can be treated only with difficulty. It is very important to be careful both about 'drag', and severe compression with your finger and thumb tips over superficial veins which may be becoming varicose. See Fig. 5.23 for the hand positions.

The tendocalcaneous can be wrung using the thumb pads and the pads of the index and middle fingers (Fig. 5.25). The basic, alternating pressures are performed on the tendon being careful not to slip into the coulisse (the hollows between the tendon and the malleoli) on each side.

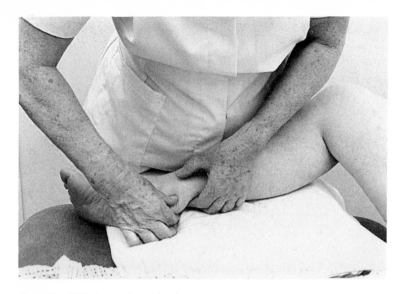

Fig. 5.25   Wringing to the tendocalcaneous.

Muscle shaking

The thigh

The rectus femoris and vastus intermedius can be shaken throughout their length by placing your nearest hand on the proximal end of the muscles, and working down to the level of the upper margin of the synovial pouch of the knee (Fig. 5.26a) Vastus medialis can be shaken from mid-point on the medial aspect of the thigh, working down to just above the knee.

With the model in prone lying, the hamstrings may be shaken together in the more slender subject, but in two lines of work when the muscles are bulky. For biceps femoris, your thumb should be carefully placed to the lateral margin of the muscle and your finger tips equally carefully placed on the medial margins of semimembranosus and semitendonosus.

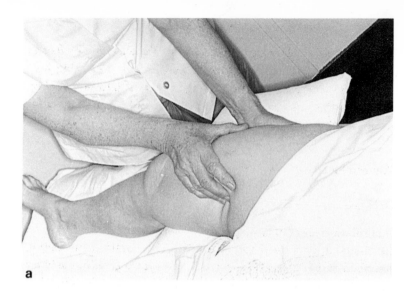

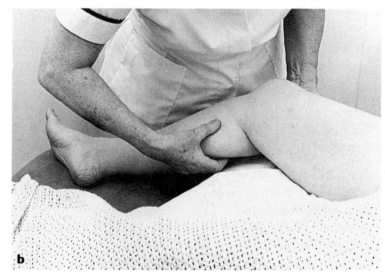

Fig. 5.26   Muscle shaking—note the fingers and thumb are in contact—the palm is off contact. (a) The thigh (b) the calf.

The calf

The whole of the calf muscle bellies may be shaken either by flexing the knee a little, and rolling the lower limb laterally then using your inside hand (Fig. 5.26b) or by turning the model into prone lying, supporting the lower leg and foot on pillows and, again, using your inside hand to perform the shaking manipulation.

Skin rolling and skin wringing

The knee

Skin rolling over a small range may be performed, and is useful, on the tissues round the knee (Fig. 5.27.) The basic manipulation described on pp. 18—19 is adapted to be performed with the index and middle fingers on one side, and the flat thumbs on the other. It is uncomfortable when performed with too great depth or over too

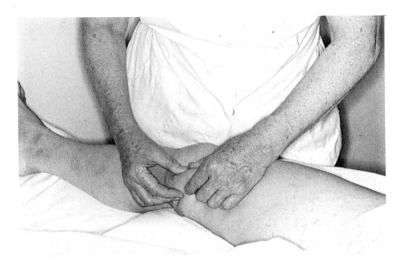

Fig. 5.28 Wringing the skin round the knee.

great a distance. It is, however, a most useful manipulation when disease or trauma has caused the structures round the knee to thicken.

Skin wringing may also be performed for similar reasons, and may be more tolerable if small areas of skin are lifted and wrung (Fig. 5.28).

Hacking and clapping

Hacking and clapping on the lower limb are usually performed regionally. Both manipulations can be completed on the thigh before proceeding to the calf and follow the petrissage to the thigh before kneading is practised on the calf.

The lines of work should go up and down the limb, with the hands striking the muscles across their length and so across the long axis of the muscle fibres.

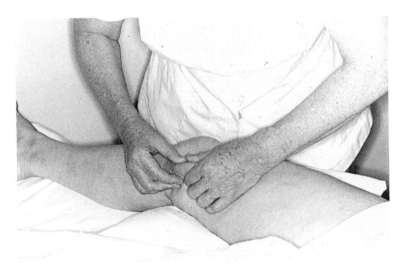

Fig. 5.27 Skin rolling round the knee using thumb and two fingers.

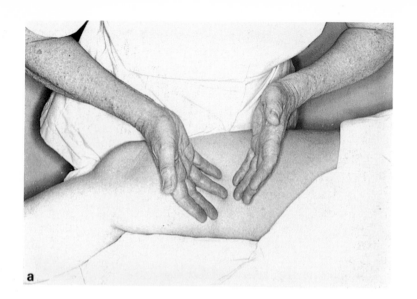

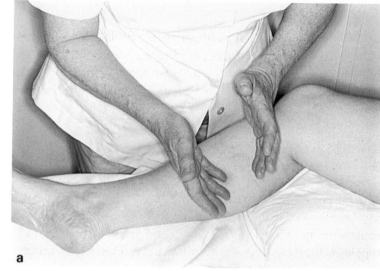

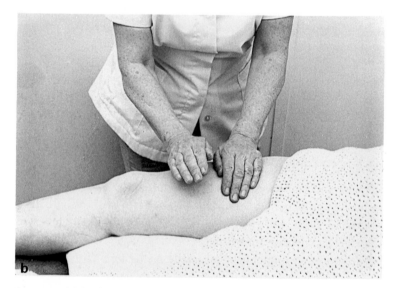

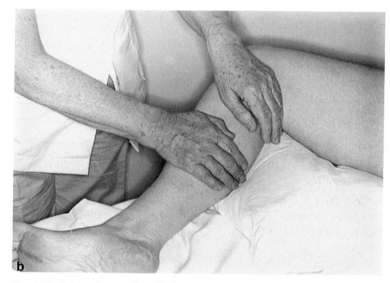

Fig. 5.29 (a) Hacking to the thigh. (b) Clapping to the thigh.

Fig. 5.30 (a) Hacking to the calf. (b) Clapping to the calf.

The thigh

For the quadriceps, start at mid-thigh on the medial side and work down vastus medialis to the knee, work to the front and continue up rectus femoris to the groin. Then move laterally to work down vastus lateralis by bending your hips and knees, after taking one pace back to get better access; then reverse along these lines (Fig. 5.29).

The bony point to avoid is the adductor tubercle, and bulky muscles may need zig-zag lines of hacking to effect complete cover.

The hamstrings are more accessible with the model in prone lying as for the petrissage manipulations. Medial and lateral lines of work may be necessary working down and up semimembranosus and semitendonosus together and then biceps femoris, in each case stopping before reaching the myotendinous junctions when hacking.

The calf

The calf muscles are usually hacked and clapped by turning the whole lower limb into lateral rotation and slightly bending the knee. Work only on the muscle bulk and avoid the tendocalcaneous. Take care when hacking to avoid any varicosed vessels (Fig. 5.30).

The anterior tibial and peroneal muscles

The anterior tibial and peroneal muscles are best treated by medially rotating the whole limb, more so for the peronei when you may also need to step further back with one leg, and bend your hips and knees to allow your forearms to be parallel with the limb. Work down to just above the level of the lateral malleolus in each case, and more lightly as the muscle bulk diminishes.

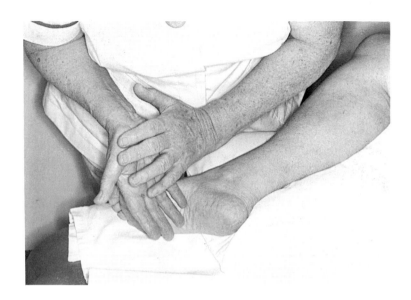

Fig. 5.31 Hacking to the foot.

The foot

Hacking on the foot is only possible on the plantar aspect of the area of the medial longitudinal arch (Fig. 5.31), and sometimes the anterior transverse arch. Both hands can be used on the former, working with the whole limb laterally rotated to give better access. One-handed hacking can be performed on the forefoot in the anterior transverse arch, with your hand working across the line of the arch.

Clapping is best performed with one hand on the dorsal and the other on the plantar aspect of the foot working simultaneously.

Chapter 6: Massage to the Back, Gluteal Region and Neck

The back and neck may be conveniently divided for treatment. The lumbar and thoracic regions are usually treated together as the 'back', but the cervical region is usually included with them for sedative treatments. The gluteal region is usually treated alone, but the lumbar region may be included with it. For treatment of the neck, the area exposed usually extends from the occiput to the lower thoracic region, so that the whole of the trapezius may be included in the treated area.

For massage to the thoracolumbar region

Preparation of the model

Ask the model to remove all clothing except briefs/pants and in the case of the female, the brassière.

Preparation of the treatment couch

Cover the couch with an underblanket and cotton sheet and fix them in position using straps. If the couch has a nose piece remove it; if not, place two pillows crossing one another at right angles at the head of the couch, so that the model's nose can rest at the crossing. Provide a small pillow to go under the abdomen and possibly one to go under the ankles. Have ready a cotton sheet to cover the body and two blankets—one large one for the trunk and legs, and a small blanket or sheet folded to go across, *under* the model's chest. When the model lies down, this blanket should be under the breasts and, in

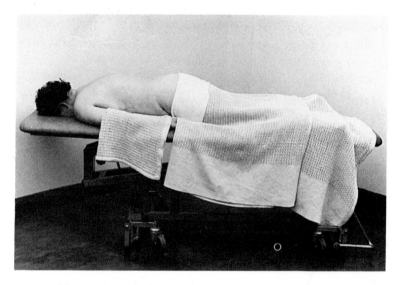

Fig. 6.1 The position of model and blankets for massage to the thoracolumbar region.

the case of the female can be held together over the upper back when the brassière is undone and while the brassière straps are removed from the shoulders. The brassière can then be pulled out from under the model without exposing her. The outer flaps of this blanket can then be used to cover the arms (Fig. 6.1). Turn the sheet and larger blanket down together, so as just to expose the upper part of the gluteal cleft. Then tuck the sides of the covers under the model's hips, so that the sheet and blanket are very firm and cannot be easily moved (Fig. 6.1).

Examine the area

Check by observation the state of the skin and posture, especially check that the axilla and groin are accessible. Ask the model to abduct both arms slightly so that you can insert your hands in the axilla to check if perspiration is excessive. If so, apply talcum powder. The pillow under the abdomen helps to create a triangular space to give access to the area above the groin. Slide your fingers round the sides to check that you can insert your fingers into this space (Fig. 6.3).

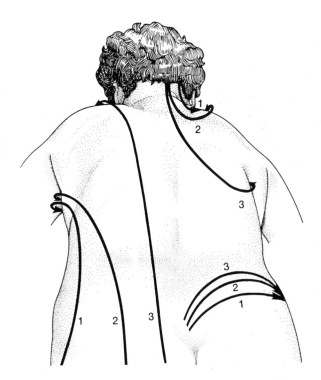

Fig. 6.2   The lines of effleurage for the lumbar, thoracolumbar and neck area.

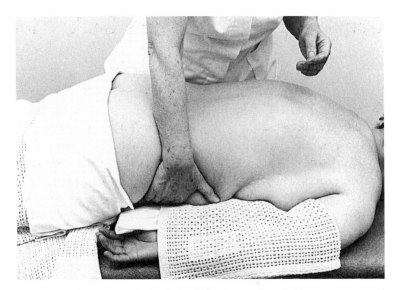

Fig. 6.3   Back massage—the finish for the lumbar strokes of effleurage.

Effleurage to the back

The back can be divided into three overlapping areas for effleurage (Fig. 6.2). Neck effleurage is directed to the supraclavicular and axillary spaces, back effleurage to the axillary space, and lumbar effleurage to the groin. It is more usual to work bilaterally and simultaneously. Stand in walk standing at the level of the model's lower thighs and lean your trunk sideways so that you can exert equal hand pressure. Your shoulders should be parallel with the model's shoulders.

The lumbar strokes start with your hands on the middle of the lumbar region at its lowest point and finish as in Fig. 6.3, at the groin, with your fingers inserted into the space by their full length. About three strokes should be made, each with an upward curve so that the whole lumbar region is treated (Fig. 6.2).

The back strokes also start with your hands in the lumbar region.

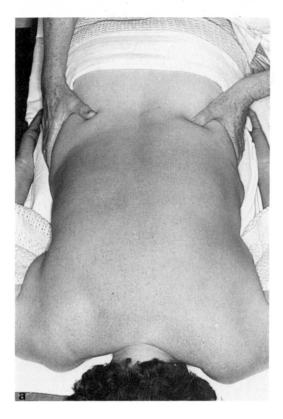

Fig. 6.4 Back massage: (a) the start of the most lateral stroke of effleurage. (b) the finish of the most lateral stroke of effleurage.

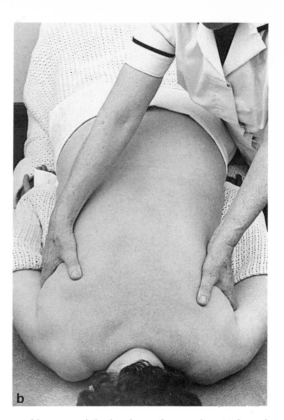

The first stroke at the sides goes to the axilla (Fig. 6.4a and b). The second stroke goes from the more central area also to the axilla (Fig. 6.5a and b). In both cases your fingers should go into the space by their full length. The third stroke proceeds up the middle of the back to the supraclavicular area, curving over the middle of the upper fibres of trapezius (Fig. 6.6).

In all cases, ensure your hands lie obliquely on the back until the appropriate space is reached when the stroke is terminated with the fingers leading. If you lead the strokes up the back with your finger tips your hands will be prevented from conforming to the hollows and humps of the back, and may also stick and make jumpy strokes. Each stroke finishes with overpressure and a slight pause at the space.

Kneading

On the back

Kneading on the back involves keeping your hands much flatter than on the limbs, yet they must curve to the part. The pressure is directed towards the axilla on the main part of the back in an upward and

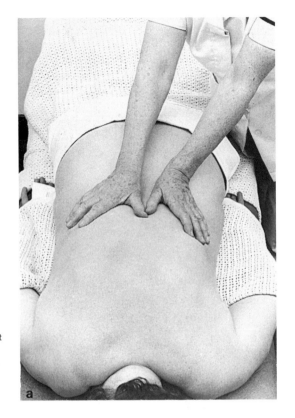
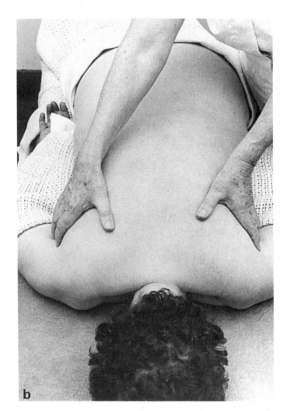

Fig. 6.5 Back massage: (a) the start of the two medial strokes of effleurage. (b) the finish of the second stroke of effleurage.

outward direction (Fig. 2.4a). Take care that your pressure is such that the depth treats the soft tissues. Poor direction of pressure can cause either uncomfortable compression of the trunk, or equally uncomfortable movement of the body either up and down, or from side to side on the support.

Alternate, double handed kneading

The lines of work proceed downwards from:
1 just below the axilla to the outside of the buttocks
2 over the scapula to the buttocks
3 over the superior angle of the scapula to the buttocks
Work in three straight lines. A narrow back will be adequately treated with two lines of work and, obviously, a broad back may need four lines of work. Each line should overlap that adjacent by half a hand width.

Your own standing position should be walk standing, with the outer leg forward and your inner hip against the couch at about the level of the model's thighs or knees. As you work down the back,

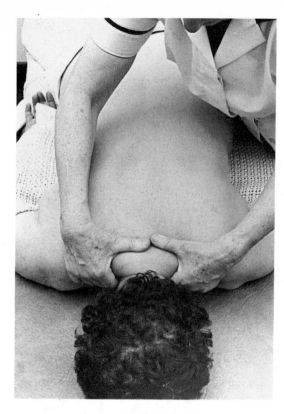

Fig. 6.6 Back massage: the finish of the third stroke of effleurage.

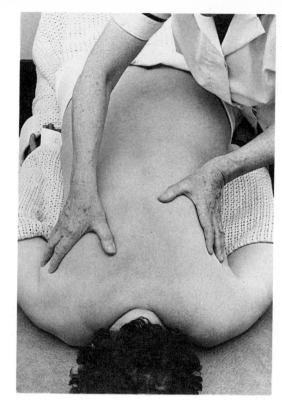

Fig. 6.7 Kneading on the back. Note the obliquity of the hands and the size of the circle. The two hands are at the maximum points of their circles from each other.

you should transfer your weight from your forward to your rear leg by gradually easing your touching thigh down the couch. In order to use your hands with even weight, lean your trunk sideways across the bed, so that both elbows are nearly equally flexed and kept like that (Fig. 6.7).

As you perform the kneading, you will find that it is necessary to start with your hands slightly oblique to the long axis of the back, and to increase the obliquity as you proceed down the back, so that on the lumbar region your hands may lie almost horizontally. This

change in hand position is essential for maintaining full hand contact (Fig. 6.7), and to allow you to work more deeply on the lumbar area. It is more usual to work with alternate hands, but more depth or more sedative work may be performed using both hands simultaneously; take care, however, not to cause the model's body to move up and down on the couch.

Do not be tempted to work at the upper back with straight elbows—this causes the whole model to move up and down on the couch.

Single handed kneading

Single handed kneading can be performed on any area of the back. It is usual to stand in walk standing facing across the couch, and either hand may be used. Keep your other hand in firm contact, ready to change hands as you tire or as you work on another area.

Superimposed kneading

Superimposed kneading is performed for a greater depth effect than single handed work. One hand is placed over the other as in Figs. 6.8 and 6.9, and the under hand maintains the contact and pressure up and out towards the axilla, but both hands provide the depth which is transmitted from your feet.

Stand in walk standing facing across the back to treat the opposite side (Fig. 2.1), and in walk standing obliquely to the couch to treat the nearside (Fig. 2.2). On the opposite side the fingers of both your hands point outwards (Fig. 6.8) and circle clockwise. On the near side your deeper hand should point outwards re-inforced by your other hand placed in the opposite direction (Fig. 6.9), and circle anti-clockwise. The lines of work are usually from:

• the axilla to the buttock
• over the scapula to the buttock

Some people prefer always to work from proximal to distal, sliding the hands up the back to restart. Others, work in a continuous line which starts under the far axilla, goes down to the far buttock, slips medially and goes up to the far scapula, slides across mid-line and reverses direction of work down to the adjacent near-side buttock and up the nearside from buttock to axilla. When this type of work is performed, difficulty may be experienced with progressing *up* the back without dragging on the second and fourth lines. The trick is to perform the circle and pressure, then release your pressure allowing the skin and subcutaneous tissues you have

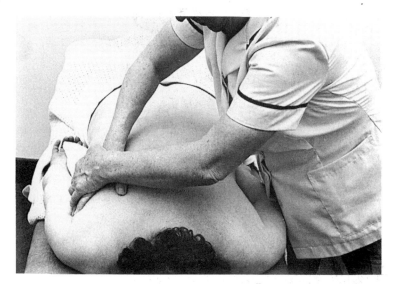

Fig. 6.8　Superimposed kneading—the far side.

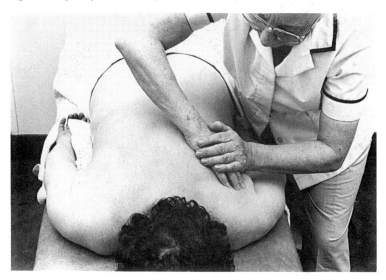

Fig. 6.9　Superimposed kneading—the near side. Note the practitioner's total change of position of feet, body and hands.

moved upwards to slide down under your hands as you start the next circle and re-apply pressure.

Thumb kneading

Stand in walk standing facing the head of the couch.

Single or double handed, alternate thumb kneading may be performed locally to any area of the back. Your thumbs are used as flat as possible, and your finger tips should rest on the back to act as a pivot but not at a depth to perform work (Fig. 6.10).

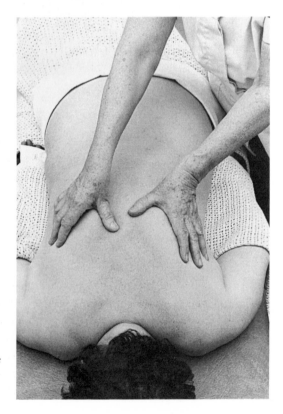

Fig. 6.10 Thumb kneading on sacrospinalis—right thumb working and left relaxing. Note their obliquity and the bulge of tissue on the outer side of the right thumb.

The area most often given thumb kneading is the length of the sacrospinalis. One thumb works on each side of the spinous processes, and the thumbs should circle round one another (not be lifted off) to move onwards. Again, use a proximal to distal sequence, starting at mid-scapular level and continuing to upper sacral level. Reach forward to start and transfer your weight backwards as in doing the alternate handed kneading.

Finger kneading

Stand in walk standing facing the direction of work.

Finger kneading is again, more usually performed on sacrospinalis, with the fingers of each hand on each side of the spinous processes. The finger pads are used, and greater depth is achieved if you tuck your thumbs into your palms rather than using them for support.

Localized finger pad kneading may be performed to any area such as the margins of the scapula, or specific muscles in the second layer of the back—e.g. the rhomboids or the levator scapulae. In this case, always work from the margins of the muscle inwards towards its main muscle bulk (Fig. 6.11), and change direction of your stance as needed.

Skin rolling—back and gluteal region

Stand in walk standing facing across the couch.

The technique described on pp. 18—20 is applicable to the back, which is dealt with one side at a time (Figs. 2.19—2.22). The lines of work are the same on each side except that on the side further away from you, work from mid-line to the side, and on the near side you may roll the skin from the side towards mid-line, but some people prefer to perform the manipulation by pulling from mid-line to the sides by lifting the skin with the thumbs, and thus reversing the performance (Fig. 6.12).

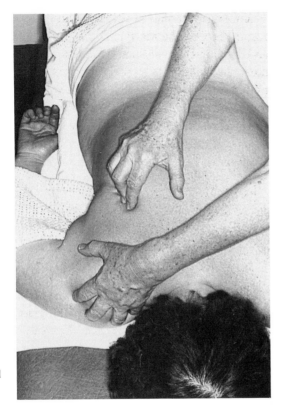

Fig. 6.11 Finger kneading round the margins of the scapula. The left hand is stabilizing the scapula.

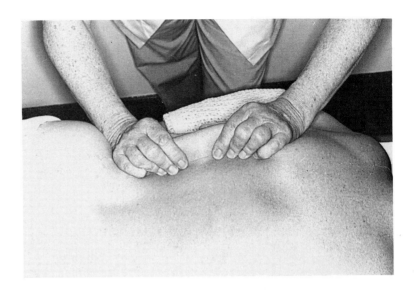

Fig. 6.12 Skin rolling—the near side.

The lines of each rolling of the skin start from the lateral end of the spinous process of the scapula and proceed to below the axilla. The lower lines of work are horizontal from mid-line to the side. On the near side you work from the side to mid-line in straight lines, until the area below the axilla is reached when the lines spread towards the spine of the scapula. Thus, on the far side you work down the back and up the back on the nearside.

In a similar way, short lines of work can be used over the shoulders from near the acromion of the scapula to the base of the neck, working forwards from the scapular spine and from mid-line

to the front and sides on each side of the neck. However, if there is considerable subcutaneous fat, the model/patient may find skin rolling in this area somewhat uncomfortable. The lines of work should be close enough together to achieve an effect on all the skin, not just on a few lines of skin.

Skin wringing

Stand in walk standing facing across the couch.

Skin wringing is not an optional manipulation to skin rolling. It is less conducive to production of a good erythema. Use it for a more mobilizing effect.

The lines of work are as those for reinforced/superimposed kneading, i.e. down and up each side of the back. The skin is lifted up by placing your hands flat on the surface as for skin rolling, then

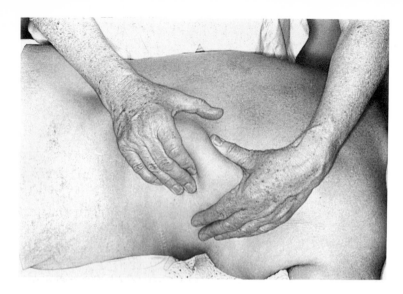

Fig. 6.13 Skin wringing.

exerting pressure with the flat fingers of one hand towards the flat thumb of the other hand (Fig. 6.13). Do not allow your hands to slide on the skin and you should obtain a roll of skin between your hands. Continuous reversal of the opposite compressing components of the hands will cause a wringing action. Do not try to work too deeply. The object is to lift and wring the superficial tissues only. Some people convert this manipulation into picking up, but the author believes that the back muscles are, on the whole, too flat to respond to such a manipulation.

Muscle rolling

Stand in walk standing facing across the couch.

Rolling of sacrospinalis is performed one side at a time. Your two thumbs form a straight line, and on the far side are placed to exert pressure outwards from between the vertebral spinous process, and the medial margin of the farside sacrospinalis. All your finger tips in a straight line should be ready to exert pressure on the margin of sacrospinalis adjacent to the rib angles/lateral processes of the vertebrae. Now, alternately push outwards and with depth with your thumbs (Fig. 6.14) and then press inwards and medially with your finger tips (Fig. 6.15). Release the pressure with each set of hand components as the other set exerts pressure and move them on to the adjacent area, so that you proceed down and then up the muscle.

On the nearside of the back, your finger tips will work on the medial margin of sacrospinalis, and your thumb lengths on the lateral margin of the muscle.

The lines can proceed from mid-scapular to the sacral region on the back.

You may be able to roll the margins of latissimus dorsi, and by careful palpation to identify and roll levator scapulae. This latter muscle is, however, more likely to need treatment with a neck condition.

Hacking and clapping

The back

Stand in walk standing facing across the couch.

Hacking and clapping on the back is done in the four lines described for kneading, i.e. two each side of mid-line, and is started under the more distant axilla.

Work down the far side, move medially and work up to below the spine of the scapula (Fig. 6.16). Jump your hands across mid-line by slightly lifting (and, in the case of hacking, pronating them more) stepping one pace backwards to do so, and continue down the medial line on the nearside of the back, then up again to the axilla.

If you wish to include the neck in the lines of work, start on the far

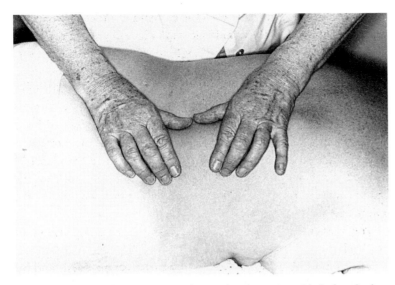

Fig. 6.14 Muscle rolling on sacrospinalis—push compression with the length of the thumbs.

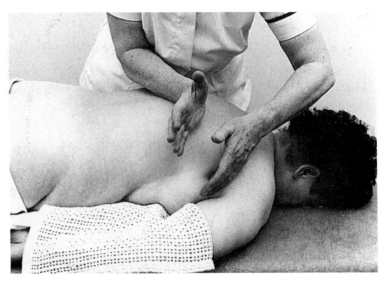

Fig. 6.16 Hacking on the back—across the fibres of latissimus dorsi.

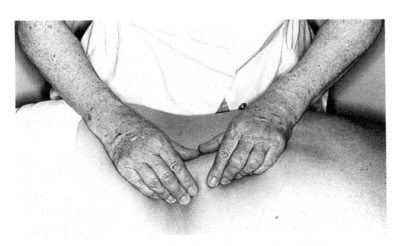

Fig. 6.15 Muscle rolling on sacrospinalis—pull compression with fingers.

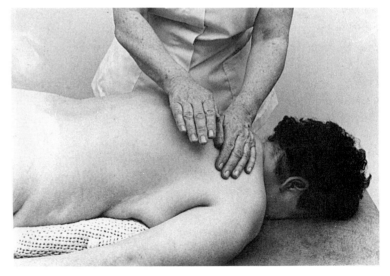

Fig. 6.17 Clapping on the back.

side of the neck and work down the upper fibres of trapezius, making a little hop over the lateral part of the spine of the scapula to continue to the axilla, and on down the back. At the near side, when you reach the axilla, you must turn your body towards your model's head and hop your hands over the spine of the nearside scapula to work up the nearside of the neck.

Clapping on the back should have a similar depth over all areas, but be lighter on the neck (Fig. 6.17).

Hacking should vary in depth so that the more bony areas have lighter treatment than those that have more soft tissue bulk, where the work should be deeper.

The gluteal region

Some practitioners treat both buttocks at once, but the model/patient may suffer discomfort as bilateral work tends to separate the gluteal cleft. Much deeper work is also feasible if one side is treated at a time.

Preparation of the model

A similar arrangement to that for the back is used, but the under-chest blanket will not be needed.

To expose only one buttock, stand on the opposite side of the prone model, grasp the covers with both hands, one each at the upper and lower levels of the buttock and lift them towards you, turning the central part between your hands over as you do so. In this way, an oblong area is uncovered with the covers pleated on each side of the exposed area.

Effleurage

Three effleurage strokes are usually performed, each finishing at the groin. It is very important not to pull the buttocks apart which is

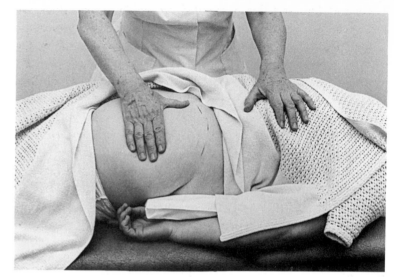

Fig. 6.18 The glutei—effleurage—starting position. The thumb is on the cross marking the posterior superior iliac spine and is pivoting to stroke along the iliac crest.

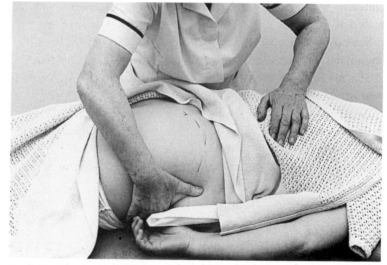

Fig. 6.19 The glutei—effleurage—the finish of all the strokes.

uncomfortable, and this is avoided by making every effleurage stroke curve. The first stroke is started with your hand nearest the model's feet on the middle of the buttock and your thumb on the posterior, superior, iliac spine—marked by the dimple (Fig. 6.18). Pivot your hand so that your thumb strokes round the whole iliac crest, then adduct it to meet your palm and continue to stroke down and out until the fingers can curve under the body to above the groin (Fig. 6.19). The next two strokes curve, respectively, with an upward arc and a downward arc, from the same mid-point of the buttock to the same point above the groin. When the model is lying with a pillow under the abdomen, there is a triangular gap formed by the upper thigh, the lower abdomen and the support. This is the groin—immediately above the superior border of the femoral triangle.

Kneading

As in performing effleurage, it is more usual to treat each side of the gluteal region separately. Kneading to this region is performed in walk standing facing the couch. The opposite buttock is treated.

Start by thinking of two or three lines of work which follow the lines of the main muscle fibres, which have an oblique direction from above medially to below laterally. Place one hand, usually that nearest the feet, so that it lies across the muscle fibres and over gluteus minimus and gluteus medius (Fig. 6.20), and work down and out towards their insertions on the upper extremity of the femur. Next, move your hand, still oblique, to the origin of gluteus maximus on the iliac crest and work down and out to the fascia lata. Repeat if necessary for a third, more medial line of work.

Superimposed kneading

Superimposed kneading should be used when the muscle bulk is great, using exactly the same lines of work. The kneading manipula-

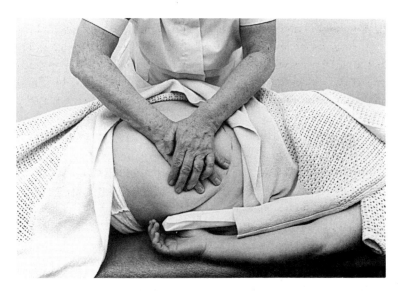

Fig. 6.20 The glutei—kneading—note the contact hand lies across the muscle fibres.

tion, in both single handed and superimposed work, is done in such a manner that the pressure is on to and through the glutei, and with great depth in the second and third lines of work, but on the more lateral line the pressure is directed inwards as though pulling towards yourself.

Frictions

Circular frictions

Circular frictions can be performed on selected areas to achieve local, deep effects. The margin of the iliac crest over aponeuritic structures giving rise to the muscles is an area sometimes needing attention. Use your unsupported thumb or fingers and gradually encroach inwards to the area of discomfort or disruption (Fig. 6.21).

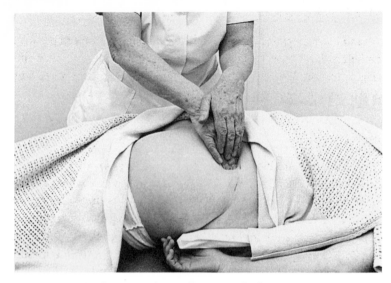

Fig. 6.21   Circular frictions to the attachments on the iliac crest.

Picking up

Work in the same oblique lines along the length of the muscle fibres as used for kneading. Stand in walk standing, using your body weight by transferring your weight forwards and backwards to exert deep pressure on the pressure phase of the picking up manipulation. Your hands will thus also have a maximum span, so that the muscles can be lifted and squeezed more easily (Fig. 6.22). The lines of work are short, and you can work up and down the muscles using single-handed, alternate picking up.

Wringing

Wringing may be feasible on some subjects. Your position and lines of work are as for picking up but the muscle bulk is passed between your hands once it has been lifted by exerting pressure with all the

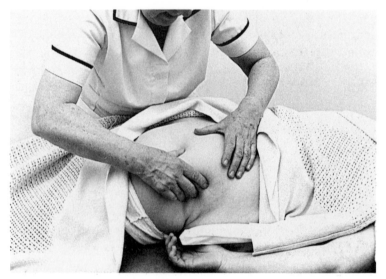

Fig. 6.22   The glutei—picking up—along the muscle fibres.

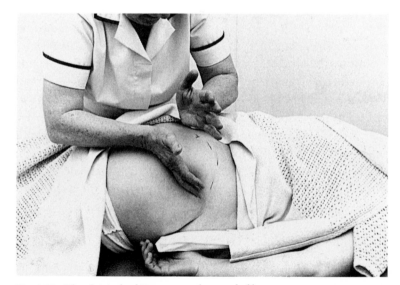

Fig. 6.23   The glutei—hacking—across the muscle fibres.

fingers of one hand and the thumb and thenar eminence of the other hand at the same time.

Hacking and clapping

The lines of work are as for the kneading so that your hands strike at right angles to the length of the muscle fibres. Hacking and clapping (Fig. 6.23 and 6.24) can both have considerable depth, but very bulky tissues may need beating or pounding which can be very deep without stinging and which are less uncomfortable for the operator to perform.

For massage to the neck

There are four positions for neck massage.

Model in prone lying

A similar arrangement to that for the back is used, but the main sheet and blanket are turned back to the level of the upper lumbar region (Fig. 6.1). For work in this position, stand level with the model's hips and in walk standing. Lean sideways towards the model.

Model in lying

The model lies supine with one or two head pillows. The undercovers should not be strapped down on to the couch, so that you can sit at the head of the couch and pull covers, pillows and model up the couch until the inferior angles of the model's scapulae are only just supported by the couch (Fig. 6.25). This is an excellent position in which to massage a very painful neck with much protective spasm.

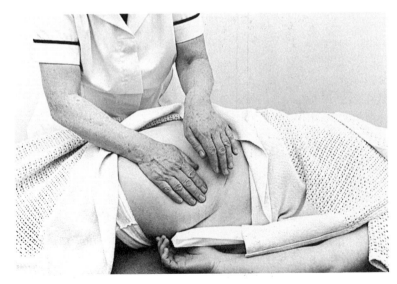

Fig. 6.24 The glutei—clapping—across the muscle fibres.

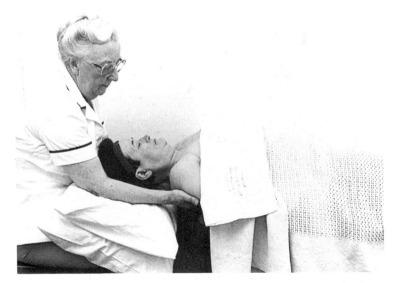

Fig. 6.25 The position of model and practitioner for treatment of the neck when it is very painful. Effleurage—neck to axilla.

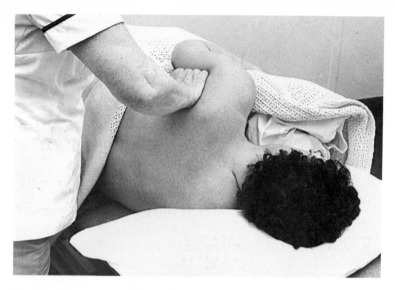

Fig. 6.26 The position of the model in side lying for treatment of one side of the neck in side lying. Effleurage—neck to axilla.

Model in side lying

The position of side lying, with two head pillows and a pillow at the front of the model to support the upper arm, can be used for unilateral work. The large blanket should be arranged to leave the upper side of the neck and the scapular region free to be massaged (Fig. 6.26). Stand behind the model in walk standing at about the level of his or her waist.

Model in forward lean sitting

Arrange a table against a wall and place on it a pile of pillows against which the model can lean with full support of his or her upper trunk, arms and head. Ask the model to sit in front of the table, preferably on a stool or a chair with a very low back (Fig. 6.27).

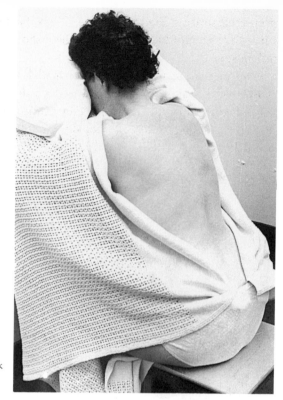

Fig. 6.27 Lean forward sitting position of the model for neck massage. Note the straight back and that the head is not flexed.

Remove the top pillow and spread a blanket on top of the pillow pile and in front of the model. The model should be already undressed except for the brassière in the case of a female. Ask him or her to place both arms on the pillow and blanket pile, leaning forward with a straight back and neck to do so. The upper corners of the blanket are then lifted, pulled across the model's arms and tucked into the model's waistband at the centre back (Fig. 6.27). In the case of a female, the brassière can then be undone and slipped off the arms. Replace the top pillow on the pile and ask the model to lean his or her head against it. If necessary, two top pillows may be crossed, as in prone lying to accommodate the nose. Check that the forward lean is still with a straight back and neck. There should especially be no neck flexion.

Stand in walk standing behind the model, and be prepared to transfer your weight forwards and backwards, and also possibly to bend your hips and knees to gain comfortable access to the thoracic region. You may, additionally, need to take a side step to each side in turn, to gain full access or better pressure for some manipulations.

Effleurage

The neck strokes are performed with the flat of the fingers starting on the sides of the neck and going to the supraclavicular glands (Fig. 6.28). A second stroke down the back of the neck, goes to the same glands, and a third stroke goes down the back and sides of the neck with more of the hand in contact, turning, over the area of the medial angle of the scapula to continue to the axilla (Figs. 6.25 and 6.26).

Similar strokes to those performed on the back should also be performed when the model is in prone lying, or lean-forward sitting (Fig. 6.28).

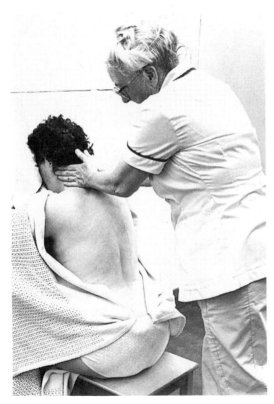

Fig. 6.28 Neck massage—the start of the more lateral stroke of neck effleurage.

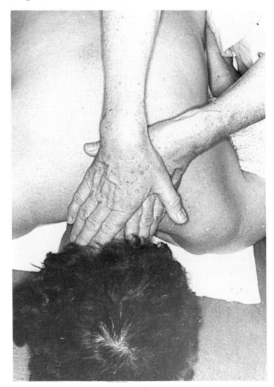

Fig. 6.29 Neck massage—kneading of the medial muscles.

When the model is in lying or side lying the lines of work are devised to follow the above patterns, bearing in mind the need for maximum hand contact and a comfortable and effective stroke, finishing at a group of lymph glands with slight overpressure and a pause.

Kneading

The neck is a difficult area as it is so confined and may be very short in some subjects. If it is treated with the model in prone lying, then the kneading may start on the neck and proceed down to whole-handed work on the wider part of the back (Fig. 6.29). As much of your hand as possible should be used for kneading, whatever the position used for the model.

The finger pads are used on the posterior aspect from the occiput (Fig. 6.29) down to where the neck widens, and then the hands are flattened, possibly overlapped, and continue on the interscapular area. On the lateral aspect of the neck, the fronts of the two distal phalanges of all four fingers (Fig. 6.31) are used until the swell of trapezius allows your whole hand to be in contact, using your palm

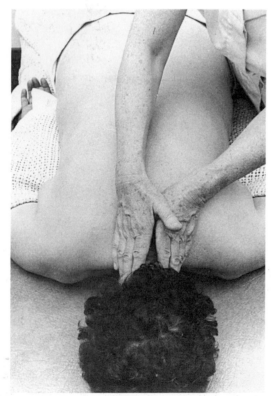

Fig. 6.30 Neck massage—kneading of the lateral muscles.

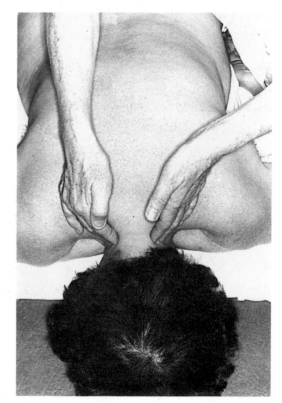

Fig. 6.31 Neck muscles—kneading of the lower lateral muscles.

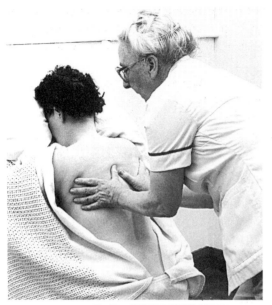

Fig. 6.32 Neck muscles—kneading continued to the middle and lower fibres of trapezius.

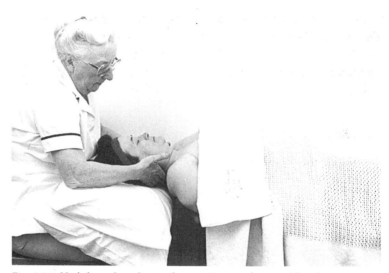

Fig. 6.34 Neck finger kneading to the posterior muscles—model supine.

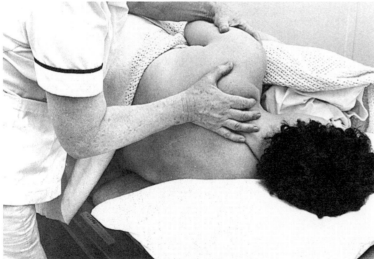

Fig. 6.33 Neck muscles—continued kneading on trapezius—model in side lying.

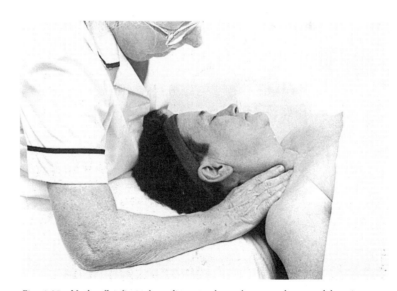

Fig. 6.35 Neck—flat finger kneading—to the scalene muscles—model supine.

MASSAGE TO THE BACK, GLUTEAL REGION AND NECK

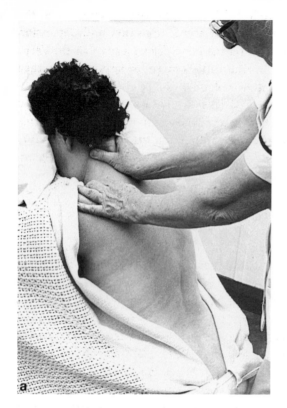

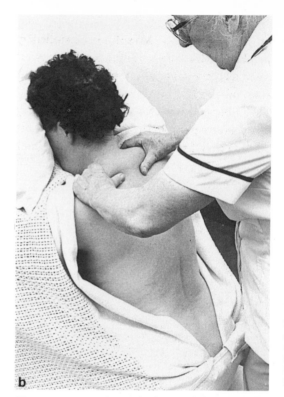

a

b

Fig. 6.36 Model in lean forward sitting: (a) a picking up type manipulation which also kneads the neck muscles. (b) continued picking up to the upper fibres of trapezius.

at the back and your fingers at the front on the upper fibres of trapezius. A squeeze knead is now performed. Flat handed kneading is performed on the upper thoracic area in a line from the interscapular area towards the axilla (Fig. 6.32).

When using your fingers, the pressure should always avoid contact with bone (the spinous and transverse processes of the upper cervical vertebrae) and should be upwards and inwards on the muscle bulk lying between the processes.

With careful adaptation of your hand the neck muscles may be treated from occipital to mid-scapular levels, and so may the upper and also middle and lower fibres of trapezius throughout their length

(Figs. 6.33—6.35). With the model supine, flat finger kneading can be performed on the scalene muscles.

Picking up

Place one hand round the whole posterior aspect of the neck and perform a single handed picking up manipulation which can evolve into simultaneous work done on the lower part of the upper fibres of trapezius with one of your hands on each side of the neck. Your fingers should be over the front of the muscle and your palms and thumbs at the back. The change from one to two handed work must be smooth (Fig. 6.36).

Muscle rolling

The posterior column of neck muscles on each side may be rolled by placing your fingers just behind the transverse processes and your thumbs alongside the spinous processes and on the same side as your fingers (as on the sacrospinalis, p.74). Work on each side in turn.

Sternocleidomastoid can be rolled in a similar manner (be very careful to exert sideways pressure only), if the model is in a suitable position (Fig. 6.37), but you may find it more feasible to put your index and ring finger tips one on each side of the muscle, and roll it by small supination and pronation movements.

Scapula rolling

If a neck is stiff and painful, it often causes the scapula to be held in abnormal postures. When the unilateral treatment technique is used,

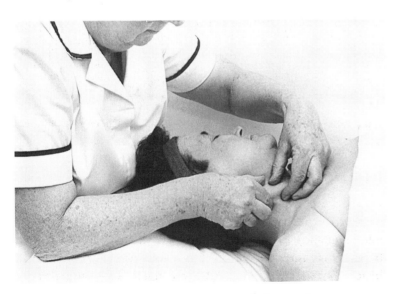

Fig. 6.37 Model supine—neck—wringing to sternocleidomastoid.

the scapula can be 'rolled'; That is, passively taken through the movements of protraction, elevation, retraction and depression while pressure is exerted on the bone. This means that the deep, scapular muscles are intermittently compressed against the rib cage with potential effect on their blood flow.

Grasp the model's arm with your arm which is nearest to the model's head, so that the forearm is comfortably supported on your forearm. Apply pressure to the scapula with your other hand. Now, circle the scapula through all four of its movements to the maximum possible range (Fig. 6.38).

Hacking and clapping

Hacking and clapping may be performed on the neck alone, with the lines of work starting near the occiput and proceeding to the lateral part of the shoulder. Two lines may be used—one more lateral, and one more posterior on the neck. The more lateral line would continue on the anterosuperior part of the upper fibres of trapezius, while the more posterior line would continue on the posterior part of the same muscle fibres. Lines of work extending on to the upper thoracic region follow the lines described on pp. 75—76

In clapping the neck, it may be necessary to work mainly with the flat fingers and be careful not to *sting*. (*Listen* for stinging—the sound is sharp.)

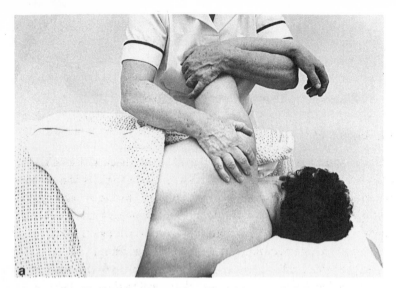 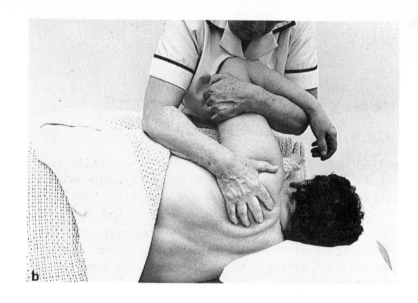

Fig. 6.38 Model in side lying—scapular rolling: (a) protracted, (b) retracted.

Chapter 7: Massage to the Face

Massage to the face

Facial massage is usually given with the model in lying, and he or she should be given a pillow under the knees, as well as pillows under the head. The practitioner will be more comfortable, and have better access in sitting at the head of the bed with the head pillows resting on his or her knee (Fig. 7.1). This position allows the practitioner's forearms to be supported for some of the manipulations, but check constantly as you work, that as the model relaxes, the head does not 'sink' into the pillow causing the neck to extend and the face to tilt.

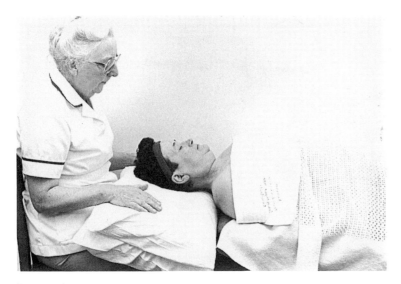

Fig. 7.1 Starting position.

Preparation of the model

Ask the model to remove outer clothing from the neck and shoulders and to remove shoulder straps. Necklaces and ear-rings should be removed as should make-up which can become smudged. Obviously, spectacles must be removed, but discuss the removal of contact lenses with the patient. If the hair is long or likely to obstruct, it can be restrained by the use of a headband.

Ask the model to lie down, and cover the body up to the subclavicular level if he or she so wishes. Ask the model to slide up the couch to rest his or her head on the pillows on your knee.

The manipulations for the face

Most of the manipulations are performed with the fingers or finger pads, and it is important to control the position of the rest of your hand, including the thumb, so that you do not rest on the patient's face.

The manipulations which may be used are:
1 effleurage
2 finger tip kneading
3 wringing
4 plucking
5 tapping
6 reverse finger tip hacking
7 vibrations to the exit foramina of the trigeminal nerve
8 finger kneading to the exit foramina of the trigeminal nerve
9 vibrations over the sinuses

10 occipitofrontalis stretching to obtain scalp movement
11 clapping to the area of platysma
12 stroke moulding to individual muscle(s).

Effleurage

Effleurage is directed from mid-line of the face to just below the ear (sub-auricular glands), taking care that as you stroke you do not constantly move the ear lobe.

As much of the palmar surface of the hand as possible is used to start the strokes. The finish is always with the finger pads, as the palms lift to clear the ear (Fig. 7.2).

The **first** stroke goes from under the chin—use your full hand (Fig. 7.3).

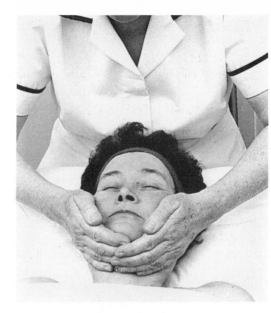

Fig. 7.3 Effleurage to the chin.

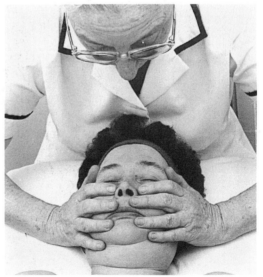

Fig. 7.4 Effleurage to the cheeks.

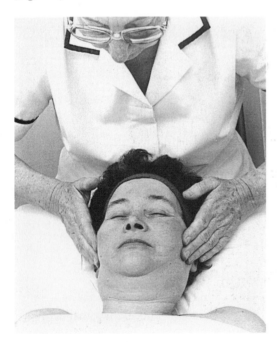

Fig. 7.2 Effleurage—the finishing position for all three strokes shown in figs 7.3, 7.4 and 7.5.

The **second** stroke starts with the fingers spread above and below the mouth—use your full hand.

The **third** stroke starts at the nose—use your finger tips to start, then your full hand (Fig. 7.4). On a small face, the **second** and **third** strokes are often combined.

The **fourth** stroke starts in mid-line of the forehead and curves downwards—use your full hand, and repeat for a **fifth** stroke if the forehead is high (Fig. 7.5).

Kneading

The lines of work are similar to those for effleurage, proceeding from mid-line to the sub-auricular area:
The first line under the chin is done with the flat of the fingers, which are also used on the cheeks to finish the next three strokes (Fig. 7.6)
Then the chin to ear line is started with the two distal phalanges
Next the upper lip to ear line is started with one finger pad
The nose to ear line is done with one or two finger pads
On the forehead two or three lines are performed with two or three finger pads (Fig. 7.7)

All the manipulations are performed with a lifting pressure upwards and inwards so that the delicate muscles are not dragged.

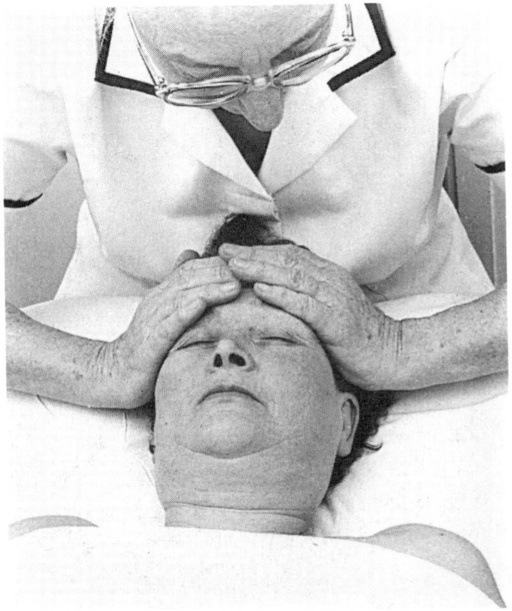

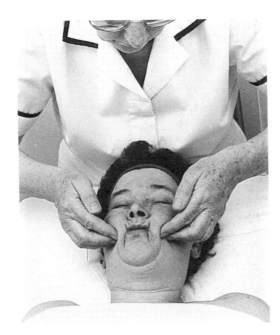

Fig. 7.5 Effleurage to the forehead.

Fig. 7.6 Kneading to the cheeks.

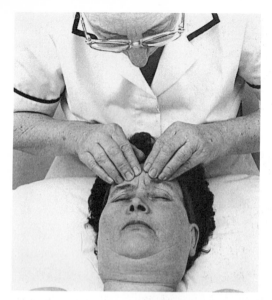

Fig. 7.7 Kneading to the forehead.

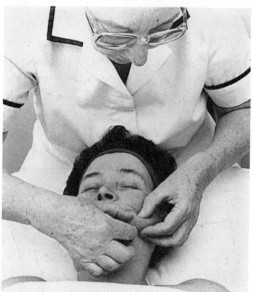

Fig. 7.8 Wrinkling to the cheeks.

Wringing

This is a finger tip wringing performed between the finger pads of the index fingers and thumbs. It is a very small manipulation. Start at the corner of the mouth and work out to the ear, then across the chin to the other ear. Now work back to the mouth, out to the ear from the nose on one cheek (Fig. 7.8) and across the forehead in three lines to the opposite ear, in to the nose and you are back at the start (Fig. 7.9).

Some people consider this manipulation should be avoided when treating facial palsy, in case the muscles are overstretched, but if the depth is light and the speed is fast, there is little reason to omit the manipulation.

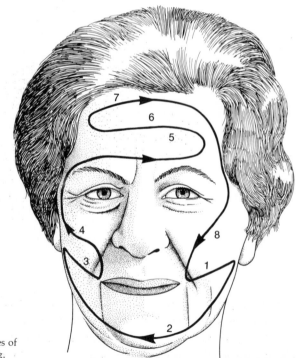

Fig. 7.9 The lines of work for wringing.

Plucking

Plucking is a stimulating manipulation performed by the tips of the thumb and index finger, in which the tissues are literally 'plucked', i.e. grasped and let go very quickly. If the tissues were held longer you would be **pinching** (Fig. 7.10).

It may be performed with one or both hands simultaneously, in similar work lines to kneading.

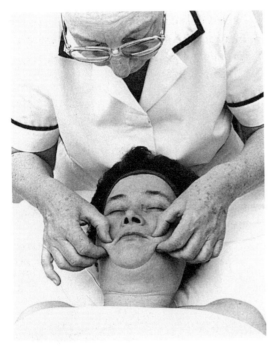

Fig. 7.10 Plucking to the cheeks.

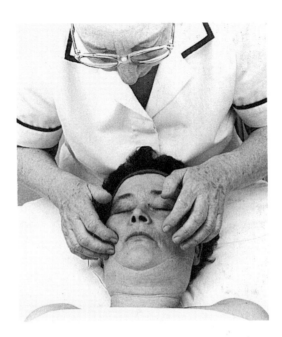

Fig. 7.11 Tapping to the cheeks.

Tapping

Tapping is performed with the finger tips (Fig. 7.11). Either one, two or three finger tips are used according to the size of the area of the face being treated. If two or more fingers are used, they may tap simultaneously, or in rapid succession as in striking two or three adjacent piano keys. The tap should be firm enough to cause slight indentation of the skin at each tap. Note that the simultaneous use of two or more fingers is likely to be heavier than sequence tapping. The lines of work are those used in the effleurage. The work may be performed on both sides of the face simultaneously, or one side of the face at a time, in which case use your other hand to stabilize the face.

Reverse finger tip hacking

Reverse finger tip hacking is performed with the palmar aspect of the medial three finger tips. The hand starts pronated and the fingers are held in slight flexion. The tissues are flicked gently with the finger tips by rapid supination of the forearm. The lines of work are those used in effleurage. The work may be performed on one side of the face or both sides simultaneously. Reverse finger tip hacking is lighter than tapping and may be used earlier when the patient is recovering from facial paralysis.

Vibrations to the exit foramina of the trigeminal nerve

Finger tip vibrations may be performed using either the index or middle finger tip over the points of exit of the ophthalmic, maxillary and mandibular divisions of the trigeminal nerve. They emerge respectively from the supraorbital notch and the infraorbital and mental foramina. The finger tip should rest lightly over the exit and constant vibrations of a small dimension are performed until discomfort diminishes. This technique is used in the treatment of both trigeminal neuralgia and tension headaches (Fig. 7.12).

Finger kneading to the exit foramina of the trigeminal nerve

The index, or middle finger tips are used to perform stationary finger kneadings over the points of exit of the ophthalmic, maxillary and mandibular divisions of the trigeminal nerve, at their respective exits through the supraorbital notch and the infraorbital and mental foramina. The finger kneadings are deeper manipulations than the vibrations described above, and are used successively with them for the same clinical circumstances (Fig. 7.12).

Vibrations over the sinuses

If the tips of your fingers and thumbs are held bunched together, and your hand is raised so that the ends of the tips rest on the skin, vibrations can be performed over a circular area (Fig. 7.13). The finger

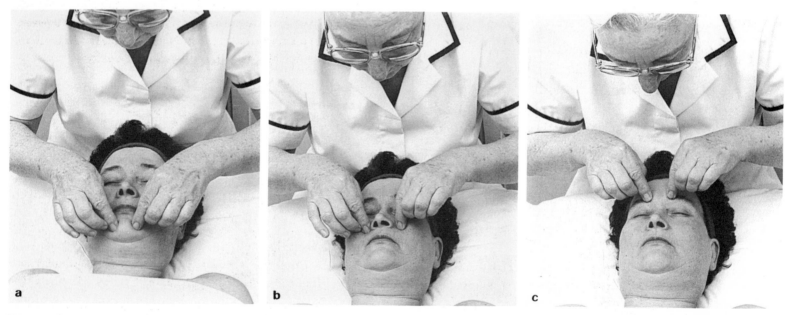

Fig. 7.12 Positions for kneadings or vibrations with one finger over the: (a) mentalis foramen. (b) infraorbital foramen. (c) supraorbital notch.

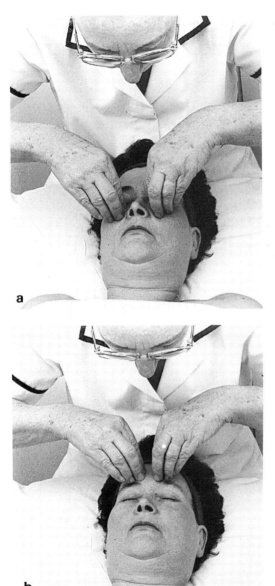

tips can be placed over the area of the frontal sinus and of the maxillary sinus, and static vibrations performed, to encourage a mechanical effect on the sinuses when they are congested and perhaps blocked. The patient can be taught to perform this manipulation, and may find that the frontal sinuses are cleared best when he or she is upright and the maxillary sinuses in the side lying position. The right sinus is drained in left side lying and vice versa.

Occipitofrontalis muscle stretching

Place the palmar surface of one hand on the forehead and the palmar surface of the other hand under the occiput. Move them simultaneously so that the hand on the forehead takes the front of the scalp downwards towards the eyebrows, and the hand on the occiput takes the back of the scalp upwards. The movement should be smooth and slow and reversed equally smoothly. The scalp will be felt to move forwards and backwards. This stretching movement is of great use in severe headache when the two bellies of the occipitofrontalis often remain in painful spasm (See Fig. 7.14).

Fig. 7.13 Vibrations with all the finger tips: (a) over the maxillary sinus. (b) over the frontal sinus.

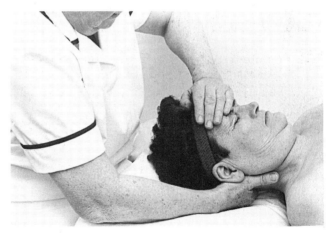

Fig. 7.14 One hand over anterior and one over the posterior belly of occipitofrontalis to rock the muscle and scalp.

Clapping to the area of platysma (Fig. 7.15)

The area below the chin can be clapped using the cupped fingers. Your hands must circle round one another in such a manner that the 'strike' is in a forward and upward direction. Be careful not to touch the front of the throat, and work at a brisk speed. The patient may learn to do this himself or herself, using the backs of the fingers.

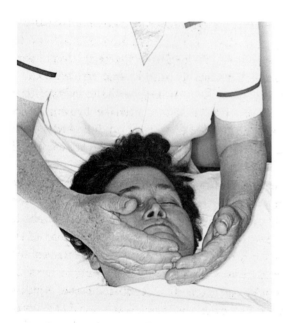

Fig. 7.15 Clapping to platysma.

Muscle moulding

Place your finger tips on each of the groups of muscles of facial expression in turn and mould the muscle actions at the same time ask the patient to attempt the muscle actions of:
• pursing the lips
• opening the mouth
• producing a mirthless grin
• smiling
• sniffing
• wrinkling the nose
• scowling
• raising the eyebrows
• closing the eyes
• blowing or whistling
• expressing disgust.

Chapter 8: Uses and Modification of Massage for Treatment

Treatment of facial paralysis or facial palsy

The paralysed muscles of facial expression are treated by using unilateral effleurage, kneading, plucking, reverse hacking and tapping. The normal side of the face should be supported with one hand covered with either a tissue or layer of cotton. Place your little finger on the chin, your ring finger on the upper lip and your middle and index fingers on the cheek with your thumb on the forehead. Apply a slight downwards and medial pressure towards mid-line of the face, and maintain it while giving the massage to the paralysed side.

Additional manipulation—eye closing

Place one forefinger along the upper eyelid and gently close and open it several times. This manoeuvre helps to lubricate the eyeball. Teach the patient to perform this manipulation.

Connective tissue massage

Connective tissue massage is a very specialized technique, first used on herself by Elizabeth Dicke of Germany. The work done by the Germans resulted in the method known as connective tissue massage and fully described by the late Maria Ebner FCSP—see Bibliography.

Briefly, the technique aims at mobilizing the deep, reticular layer of the dermis where the gel-like, ground substance is found, and is strongly related to the multiple links between the autonomic and somatic systems.

This system is dependent on thorough examination of the patient in sitting as in Fig. 8.1, starting with inspection of the back to identify alterations in contour, due to flattening or elevation caused by the changes in other structures supplied by that dermatome.

Manual examination follows, to investigate the mobility of the various layers of connective tissue, and the tension present in the muscular layers. A pattern of examination is followed which includes lifting and stroking manipulations along the paravertebral area.

The manual technique used for treatment is performed with the middle finger, using either the tip or the finger pad extending the length of the distal phalanx on the radial side. Moderate touch is applied to the patient's skin to obtain adherence (never use lubricants), and the middle finger is supported by the distal phalanx of the ring finger. The fingertip is applied at an angle of 45° to the skin (Fig. 8.1), and the slack is taken out of the superficial tissue. A pull is exerted in the direction of the desired stroke, with the radial or anterior side of the wrist joint leading, so that the superficial connective tissue is moved on the deeper connective tissue. A ripple of skin should move before the stroking finger. The patient should feel only a sensation of touch, or a slight scratching or cutting sensation. More severe sensations may indicate a need for revision of technique by:

- varying the speed of the stroke
- shortening the stroke
- varying the depth by altering the angle of the hand (decrease in the

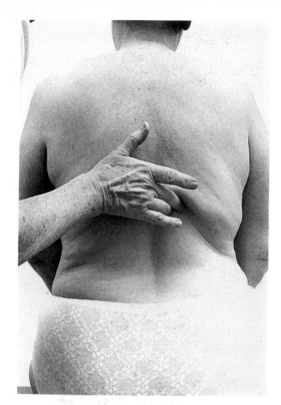

Fig. 8.1 Position and technique for connective tissue massage.

angle decreases the depth, and increase in the angle increases the depth).

The strokes are performed in the lines of the dermatomes, towards the mid-line in the paravertebral areas and in the direction of the muscle fibres in peripheral areas.

On the back, the right side is treated with the practitioner's right hand and the left side with the practitioner's left hand. On the periphery, the appropriate hand to the practitioner's position in relation to the patient is used. Ebner stresses that the appropriate paravertebral dermatomes should always be treated before the peripheral work is undertaken.

Evacuation of secretions from the chest

(Practise this first on a model.)

Percussive manipulations and vibrations are used to assist patients to evacuate secretions.

The percussive manipulations

Any of the percussive manipulations may be used to help to remove secretions and they should usually be performed over a thin covering to reduce skin effects. They are frequently combined with **postural drainage** so the patient should first be placed in the pre-determined drainage position which should, if possible, allow you to see the patient's face. Cover the area to be treated with a thin blanket or single layer of sheet or towel and ensure it is smooth (Fig. 2.32). Warn the patient the treatment is likely to be noisy and will be deep. Try to stand in such a position that the patient cannot breathe on you.

Clapping is performed by placing one or both hands in position and initiating the deeper clap described on p. 24 (Figs. 2.31 and 2.32). Clap more lightly than your planned eventual depth. Gradually, work more deeply and try to intersperse your work with encouragement to the patient to cough by using long, expiratory breaths or by huffing.

Over the smaller areas, such as the apices of the lungs, single handed work may be all that is possible. Double handed work is feasible over the area of the lower lobes of the lungs, and your hands may be able to move forwards and backwards on the lower rib cage. The depth effect you should try to obtain is that of slight jarring of the chest. It is sometimes likened to the sharp blows struck on the bottom of a newly started, or nearly empty sauce bottle. Think of trying to jerk sticky secretions off the lung tissue to which they are adhering, and aim for a loosening effect.

Hacking is performed in similar areas, but allows both hands to be used in smaller areas such as over the lung apices. The depth effect is much less, but may be sufficiently effective on the very young patient, or safer on those who have a tendency to osteoporotic bones (Fig. 2.34).

Beating and/or pounding are alternatives which give your hands a rest. Beating may also give you very localized greater depth and can be used to dislodge obstructive secretions or inhaled objects. Pounding is certainly less tiring on your finger tips than hacking, and can be used on smaller areas as a variation from hacking, and to obtain more depth. The mode of performance is described and illustrated in Chapter 2, Figs. 2.36 and 2.37.

Chest vibrations

As with the percussive manipulations, the patient is placed in a pre-determined position which either enables him or her to cough more effectively, or allows gravity to assist the drainage of secretions.

One side of the chest is usually treated at a time. If the patient is very small, for example a baby, you will find the whole chest can be completely covered by your hand, but you must in such cases avoid treating both lungs at once by using only part of your hand. The smaller the chest, the more important it is that you only give vibrations and do not exert a squeeze which obstructs respiration and can cause a great increase in the heart rate.

For the apex of one lung

Place your hands, one at the front and one at the back, over the area of the lung apex. Your anterior hand should have the finger tips resting below the clavicle, and you must avoid compression of breast tissue. To this end, keep your hand oblique so that your palm is more lateral than your fingers. Your posterior hand should be at a higher level as in Fig. 8.2.

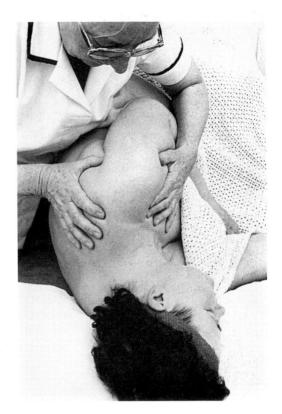

Fig. 8.2 Chest vibrations—hand positions for the apex of the lungs.

For the middle lobes of the lung (left lingula)

Place your hands, one at the front and one at the back, as in Fig. 8.3, so that your rear hand lies over the area occupied by the lower half of the scapula. If necessary, the patient's scapula can be protracted by stretching his or her arm forwards, to allow your rear hand to lie over some part of ribs 3–7. Your front hand should cover the same ribs in such a manner as to avoid the breast. Your two thumbs should be adjacent to each other in the mid-axillary line.

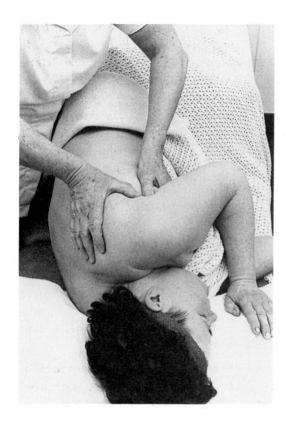

Fig. 8.3 Chest vibrations—hand positions for the middle areas of the lungs.

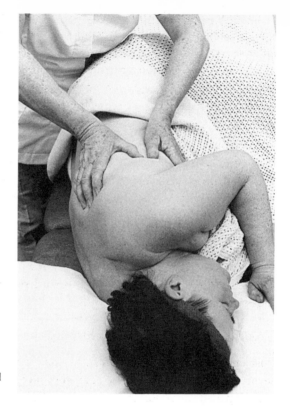

Fig. 8.4 Chest vibrations—hand positions for the basal areas of the lungs.

For the lower lobes of the lung

With your thumbs adjacent in the mid-axillary line, place your hands along the line of ribs 6–10. Your front hand should be below the breast and along the line of the costal cartilages, while your rear hand should be along the line of the ribs (Fig. 8.4).

The vibrations are first given without commanded respiratory action, but will be more effective if each burst of vibration is in time with the patient's expiration and if the burst of vibration lasts for the whole expiratory phase. You should rest on each inspiratory phase.

Initially, vibrate gently, first with one hand, then the other, then both together. The single handed work allows you to explore the patient's relaxation and rigidity of the chest wall. It also accustoms the patient to your touch and to the manipulation. As you start the double handed work, ensure that you maintain an even pressure with all parts of your hand which are in contact. Be especially careful to avoid excess pressure with the heels of your hands. Under no circumstances should your hands shake sideways, which will be ineffective.

The vibratory action must be in and out with your hands, so that you obtain a fast vibratory action of your hands towards one another, and through the patient's chest. Try to increase your depth a little as the expiration proceeds. A greater increase in depth is possible when the patient can perform active expirations as you perform the vibrations and follow the inward movement of the chest wall. At the end of the expirations, hold the compressive pressure of your hands (*Do not jerk*) for a short interval, and then release your hand pressure suddenly. The patient will breathe in. If the patient wishes to cough, you can assist by holding your pressure without vibrations. It is also most important to avoid exerting pressure which is more inclined to push the whole thorax into the bed, instead of giving pressure only through the chest wall.

The amount of inward movement of the chest wall which you can obtain will be greatest at the lung bases, and will be less at the lung apices. The range of movement will also be less in the elderly, and in those with chronic chest conditions.

Treatment of (post-operative) flatulence

Post-operative flatulence is most uncomfortable, and can cause severe discomfort to those patients who have had the abdomen or pelvis opened for abdominal, gynaecological or urological reasons, or for Caesarian section. Non-operative flatulence, which may be symptomatic of serious disorder, should be diagnosed before you attempt treatment, but simple colicky wind can be treated with good effect by giving abdominal vibrations (Fig. 2.35) with the patient in crook lying. Stand on his or her right side.

In the case of the post-operative patient, treatment can start the day after operation with gentle, single handed vibrations to the sides of the abdomen, avoiding the area of the scar. Gradually, encroach on to the central area of the abdomen so that your hand works, as far as is feasible, over each part. The depth of the vibration can be increased as the pain lessens or wind is voided.

If the patient is able to do so, he or she can place his or her hand under yours so that, as you continue the treatment he or she is made aware of how to give self vibrations. Self application can then be used as needed. However, if there are any specially painful areas, continue to give the vibrations in a stationary manner, and allow the patient to rest. As the patient becomes accustomed to the treatment, and it starts to be effective, you can start to stroke as you perform the vibrations, thus giving a labile treatment. The strokes may be performed from the left to right sides of the abdomen, or on each side from over the lower rib cage towards the iliac area.

Babies with post-feeding wind or colic may respond to vibrations performed gently over the lower back. Intersperse the vibrations with circular rubbing, with a little upward pressure over the middle of the back.

Using lubricants

Preparation

OF THE PATIENT Support the area to be treated, and ensure his or her general comfort. Spread under the area a protective, waterproof sheeting covered with either a washable sheet or towel, or a disposable sheet. Uncover the area.

OF THE TRAY This should be suitably adjacent to the area to be treated.
using lanolin—the lanolin or lanolin cream
        —a bowl of swabs
        —a receiver for dirty swabs
using oil—the oil
      —small dish or container
      —bowl of swabs
      —receiver for dirty swabs

using soap and oil—the oil

        —small dish or container

        —bowl of swabs

        —dish containing non-caustic soap

        —bowl of hand-hot water (the hottest your palm
                will tolerate)

        —receptable for dirty swabs

        —hand towel

OF THE PRACTITIONER Remove rings and wristwatch, and ensure your nails are short. Try to sit down so that you can relax and maintain a prolonged treatment without undue fatigue.

The treatment

USING OIL OR LANOLIN OR UNG. EUCERIN Open the container and leave the cap off. If using oil, pour a little into the dish.

Examine the part to be treated and using your finger or thumb tips apply the lubricant to the margins, then to the centre of the area. If possible, support your forearms or elbows adjacent to the treatment area and, using your lubricated finger or thumb tips work from the periphery to the centre of the area.

As you work, the lubricant may 'disappear' so add more, a small amount at a time, on the area on which you are at present working. Do not, at any point swamp or flood the area.

On completion, *either* leave the residual lubricant on the skin *or* gently swab most of it away, using a clean swab for each sub-section cleaned, and wiping the central area first followed by the margins.

USING SOAP AND OIL Open the container of oil and pour a little into the small dish. Put the **palmar surface only** of your hands on to the surface of the hot water, so that the dorsal surface does not become wet. Use the soap to work up a good lather on the front of your hands. Pour about 5ml (one teaspoon) of oil onto the palm of one hand, and work your palms together to distribute the oil into the lather.

Apply your hands to the area to be treated spreading the lather over the whole area. If you need more lather, repeat the above procedure, but you will find the lather spreads over a large area. Now, work with one or both hands over the whole area using stroking or kneading type manipulations. The object is not to work deeply, but to spread the lather and loosen scales of skin. As the scaly patches are loosened, use a swab to remove them from the work area.

If the lather dries up or disappears, remoisten your palms and work them together first. You may find the lather reforms, but if not recreate lather by following the above procedure.

On completion of the treatment, *either* wipe the whole area with swabs, working on a whole limb from proximal to distal, or on a smaller part from centre to periphery. This will leave a thin coat of oil on the area. *Or* wash the area by first washing your own hands and rinsing them, then lathering them so that you can apply a non-oily lather to the part to wash it. Rinse, swab clean as above, then dry the part if necessary.

Treatment of scars, burns and plastic repairs

All scars, whether primary lesions, secondary repairs or grafts, have a tendency to contract by as much as $\frac{1}{3}$ of their length. All injuries to the skin, whatever the cause also tend to become oedematous, and may become slow-healing and indurated. The oedema can be a disaster in the case of a skin graft which may be 'lifted' and prevented from 'taking' by the oedema.

At best, permanently contracted scars will cause inconvenience and at worst they cause gross deformities with severe functional limitation.

Along with other measures, the appropriate application of suitable massage techniques will help to maintain scar length and assist the movement of oedema so that it may be resolved or absorbed.

The appropriate moment at which to massage any scar, healing burn or plastic repair will be determined by the state of the healing process, the other underlying injuries or lesions and the imperative need to prevent the above complications. It must be borne in mind that over-zealous and too early massage may encourage the formation of hypertrophic (keloid) tissue to which burns victims are especially prone.

Contact materials are usually used as they lubricate the skin, allow gliding without friction and often make painful manipulations more tolerable. The different oils and their uses are explained on p. 4, and it should be noted that where wounds are still unhealed, great care must be taken to avoid infection. The selected lubricant should be sterile and renewed daily or at each treatment, and it should be used only up to the margin and not over the open wound.

The massage manipulations which are used are those suitable to treat the state at that moment. Thus, the initial or persistent oedema must be treated by clearing the venous and lymphatic vessels proximal to the wound, using the techniques described for oedema on p. 105. The localized area of oedema may need finger tip vibrations, effleurage strokes initially at the margins and gradually encroaching on to the more central area, followed by finger or thumb kneading interspersed with effleurage strokes, until the swelling is softer and the patient tolerates handling better.

Next, use as much of your hand as possible to apply pressure over a larger area (Fig. 8.5)—the central (unhealed) area may be covered with a sterile dressing and gently kneaded, maintaining even pressure and attempting to compress and move the whole scarred and swollen area. Rocking the whole area may be feasible, using your

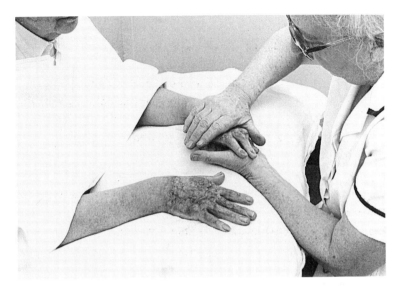

Fig. 8.5 Compressive palmar kneading to the dorsum of a burnt and grafted hand.

hands as in Muscle Rolling (Fig. 2.23). Complete your work, by effleurage strokes from distal, round the scar to the proximal lymph glands including the scar in the strokes if possible. It may be necessary to work more lightly over the scar itself with these strokes.

The scar which is less oedematous but more bound down or contracted greatly, is treated by initial, and gradually deepening, effleurage strokes round the periphery, followed by finger and thumb tip kneading to the same area (Figs. 8.6, 8.7, 8.8). Then, work on to the scar with the small kneading manipulations, continuing until the skin is either warmer to touch, or pink or both. Start slowly, and increase your speed as the patient's tolerance increases.

Now start to use stretching manipulations, which may be finger or thumb tip kneading with greater depth and slightly greater range, or stretching strokes (Fig. 8.9), working along the length of the scar, and gradually using the side of your thumb or finger to push up against the scar as you stroke along the margin.

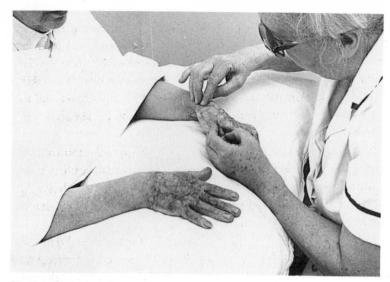

Fig. 8.6 Finger kneading to the periphery of the burnt hand.

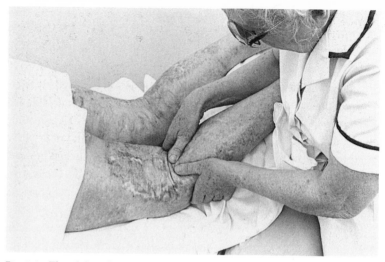

Fig. 8.8 Thumb kneading to the central and more mobile area of burns to the back of the knee.

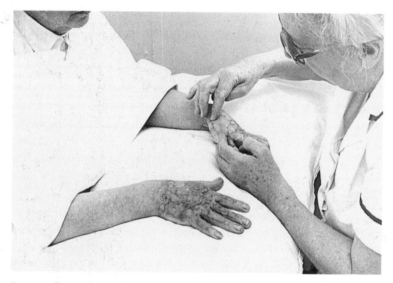

Fig. 8.7 Encroaching and deepening the finger kneading.

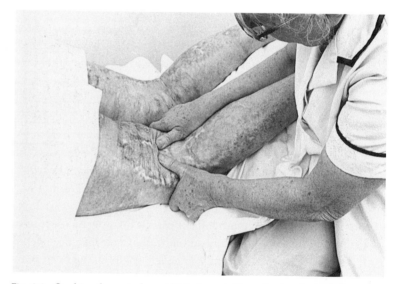

Fig. 8.9 Stroking the central area. Note the wrinkle at the thumb tips indicates some skin mobility.

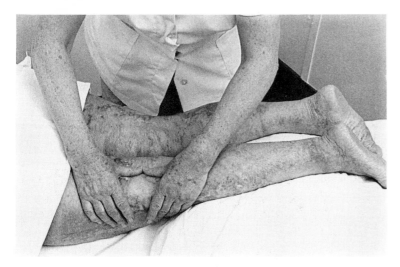

Fig. 8.10 Rocking the whole area from side to side.

Intersperse with rocking the whole scar (Fig. 8.10) along its length from side to side using either one or both hands, and then attempt small wringing manipulations (Figs. 8.11 and 8.12). Identify the worst areas and give them special attention, perform local skin wringing and skin rocking, finishing with effleurage round and to the whole area from distal to it, and up to the proximal lymph glands.

In some cases, you may find it better to support the more distal part of a limb manually and apply stretch with your supporting hand as the tissues become warm and softer (Fig. 8.13). The stretch should be so gentle as to be unobtrusive and should not make the patient aware of increased discomfort.

In the section on kneading in Chapter 2, it was stressed that the circling of the hand should avoid sudden points and becoming pear shaped. In working to stretch scars by kneading, a more pear shaped

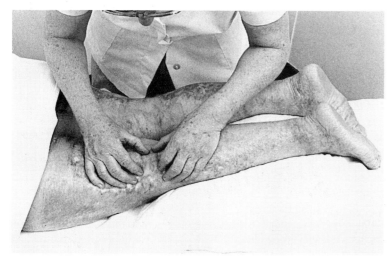

Fig. 8.11 Wringing a small area using finger and thumb tips on the back of the knee.

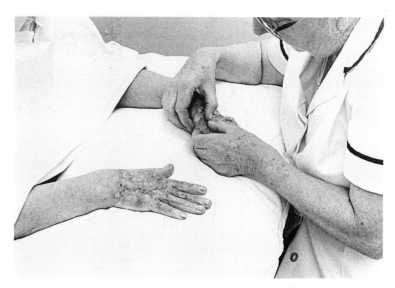

Fig. 8.12 Wringing on the side of the hand to mobilize the adherent skin.

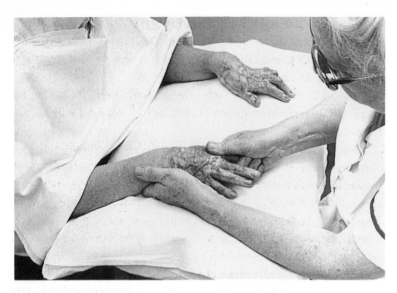

Fig. 8.13 Squeeze kneading to each finger with stretch on the tip to maintain extension.

manipulation should be cultivated. The 'point' of the pear shape, being the moment of greatest stretch on the tissues.

At the completion of the massage, the surplus lubricant may be wiped off with the swabs, or may be left on the skin to facilitate its lubrication. The patient should, if possible, be taught to use a selection of appropriate manipulations on his or her own scars.

Treatment of haematoma (bruising) or painful areas

Painful areas may be treated by massage in an attempt to relieve the pain. Areas of disorder often have local spasm which is protective. As the attempt to protect against movement of the part spreads yet more spasm will spread to the adjacent areas. Spasm prevents drainage and thus causes local congestion. Metabolites accumulate and increase the disorder and discomfort.

Bruising or haematoma are the consequence of injury, and may both present at the site of the injury, and in adjacent or distal areas into which the extravasated blood will spread. It is important to differentiate between the local haematoma at the site of the injury, which should not be treated for up to four days until damaged small blood vessels have had time to heal, and the more distant accumulation of extravasated blood, which may show as swelling as well as bruising. This oedema may be treated early to avoid consolidation, but care must be taken to cause no drag or pull on the site of the lesion. The techniques described on p. 105 should be used.

The local bruised area which may well be painful, and the painful areas described in the first paragraph can be treated in a similar manner.

Start proximal to the lesion, and clear the proximal structures using effleurage, kneading and possibly picking up.

Then work round the affected area, initially not touching it, but using stationary finger, thumb or palmar kneading, followed by small strokes of effleurage with the same hand component from the area worked upon to a more proximal normal area. If the patient will tolerate it, gradually encroach on the margins, and then the more central part, of the affected area using the same techniques. If, however, the area is very tense and painful, place as much of your hand as possible over the area and give vibrations. Keep on with the vibrations until you feel the area becoming less tense, when it may be possible to use gentle finger or thumb kneadings to the margins and work inwards.

Another useful local manipulation is gentle rocking of the area. This is especially helpful on a bruise or local swelling. Place your hand so as to encompass the whole area and gently move the mass sideways. Initially, the rocking must be gentle and not too deep, but eventually depth can be increased, and your hand can move up and down the area as in rocking, described on p. 103.

Intersperse the rocking with short strokes of effleurage and more kneading on the margins of the affected area, continuing until you feel softening of the tissues, diminution of tension and the patient experiences relief of pain. Persistent thickenings may be treated by using circular frictions with great care. Again, start round the margin and encroach to the centre and intersperse with effleurage strokes towards the nearest lymph glands.

Manipulations for the treatment of oedema

There are two extremes of oedema. That which is softer, mobile and usually of recent origin and that which is consolidated, indurated and usually of much longer standing. Oedema may present at any stage between these states. The earlier it can be treated, the better the result is likely to be.

Any restrictive clothing should be removed from the area proximal to the oedema so that drainage is facilitated. All oedematous areas should be elevated for a period of time (usually one hour) prior to massage.

The elevation should be such that the limb is supported at an angle of about 45° to the horizontal, and care must be taken that the trunk and head are not also raised causing an increase in this angle. Thus, the patient should lie as flat as possible, using pillows to support the head and not to elevate the trunk. Each part of the limb under treatment should be elevated more than the next most proximal part, to allow drainage through the increasingly large veins and lymph vessels and through the lymph glands (Fig. 5.1).

The patient should be encouraged to help during elevation, massage and afterwards, by performing a series of deep breathing exercises. The effect of a deep breath is to cause a lowering of the negative pressure in the mediasteinum, so that lymph and venous blood at a higher pressure in adjacent areas will flow to the lower pressure area.

Some massage manipulations can be combined with active contraction of the muscles under treatment, and at the end of the massage regime, active exercises should be taught with stress on slow, sustained contractions and relaxation, and regular repetition throughout the day.

The area proximal to the oedematous area, should be treated by all manipulations that will assist drainage to leave clear passage for the accumulated fluids.

Thus effleurage, slow deep kneading with extra compression, and slow compressive picking up should be performed from the most proximal lymph glands (groin or axilla) to the part where the oedema starts. Each effleurage stroke should be accompanied by a deep inspiration, both timed for maximum inspiration by the time of arrival of your hands at the appropriate group of lymph glands (space).

The treatment of the oedematous area will differ with the type of oedema but the basic rules are the same for any type of oedema. The area is treated one hand width at a time. Each hand width is constantly drained as the oedema is softened and moved so that it is included in effleurage strokes to the most proximal area.

The more proximal, oedematous area should be regarded as having four aspects like a four sided tube, and opposing aspects are handled together. Thus, aspect *one* is treated with counterpressure on opposite area *three*. Then area *three* is treated with counterpressure on area *one*. The same manipulation is performed on areas *two* and *four*, before the manipulation is changed for a deeper or more mobilizing technique. All manipulations in which the tissues are moved sideways are initially performed very slowly.

The manipulations which are of use on **soft** oedema are:

1 Vibrations performed single handed with opposite counterpressure on each aspect, followed by double handed vibrations on opposite aspects.

2 As the tissues become less tense, a very small range, stationary, single handed kneading can be performed first on one aspect, then

the opposite, then on the two sides together. Intersperse this manipulation with effleurage, and increase the size of the hand circling, as the tissue mobility increases.

3 If the oedema is in the deeper tissues, a squeeze kneading may be used. Place your two hands on opposite aspects of the part in firm, and complete contact, with your index fingers more proximal. Now exert more pressure successively with your hand in the line of the little, ring, middle and index fingers, i.e. the finger and area of palm proximal to it press together. The pressure is maintained with each component as the squeeze extends until the whole hand is exerting pressure. Thus, any fluid is squeezed onwards by the width of your hand. Effleurage again.

4 Still working in a box formation stationary, double handed kneading can be performed on all four aspects, with an increasing depth and range of manipulation.

Then, move on to the next hand width down the part and repeat the manipulations, working gradually over the oedematous area.

The ankle and foot

In spite of oedema which rounds the contours, this area presents special problems as only the sole of the foot is muscular, and the shape of the parts require special disposition of the hands.

The same manipulations are used, in the same manner and order, but one of your hands may well encompass the front and sides of the ankle, while the other treats the medial and lateral aspects of the tendocalcaneal area (often called the medial and lateral coulisse), using the length of your thumb and thenar eminence on one side, and on the other two distal phalanges of all four fingers, flexed at the proximal interphalangeal joints. In effect, a triangular plan of action should be evolved, and you should use additionally your flat fingers or palms according to the way they fit on the area under treatment.

On the foot, the sole is given constant counterpressure, as, if the patient is ambulant, the compressive force of weightbearing will stop oedema accumulating under the foot. Treatment is then directed at the dorsum of the foot and at the toes.

The wrist and hand

The more confined area of the wrist and hand, even when swollen, will require disposition of your hands in opposite directions so as to encompass the area. One hand is placed vertically on one aspect, and the other hand is wrapped horizontally round the opposite side of the limb. This hand disposition can be used for the same sequence of manipulations as on the proximal areas. Unlike the sole of the foot, the palm of the hand can become swollen and require treatment. The digits are each long enough to be squeezed using one hand on each digit, and the dorsum of the hand is usually treated initially using your palm, and eventually the length of the sides of your thumbs in the interosseus spaces.

As each area is treated, encourage active movements of the joints of that part. If necessary, demonstrate the required movement passively a few times, then require slow, active movements with a 'holding' (isometric) contraction at the end of the range in each direction. These contractions can be enhanced by a firm squeeze knead performed at the same time.

The manipulations which are of use on **consolidated** oedema are:
1 single handed kneading with as large a range as the tissue state allows. Opposite compression is essential.
2 alternate double handed kneading on opposite aspects followed by simultaneous double handed kneading
3 if any softening of tissues occur, squeeze kneading may be performed and interspersed with effleurage
Eventually, kneading may be increased in depth and range until the tissues feel softer.

Massage techniques for inducing relaxation

All massage manipulations used to induce relaxation should be performed to two rules:
1 the tempo should be slow
2 the repetition of each manipulation should continue without interruption or change until either the practitioner detects a reduction in tension, or feels the palmar surface of his or her hands becoming numbed. Thus, the patient might be equally aware of numbness.

In addition, your own movements should be smooth and rhythmical. Local relaxation techniques may be applied to any part of the body, obeying the basic rules of making the model/patient comfortable and adopting a position yourself in which you can sustain a prolonged performance of the chosen manipulation. For most areas, the manipulations to be performed would be in one of these orders:

either: *or*:
- stroking   • effleurage
- kneading   • kneading
- effleurage

The choice will depend partly on the recipient's response to stroking—some people dislike being stroked from proximal to distal—when effleurage would be substituted; and partly on the reasons for using a relaxation massage. It may be that a painful, congested area will not relax until it is decongested, when effleurage may be used first. In some cases it may even be necessary to start with stationary vibrations, followed by labile vibrations when a stroke is made as the vibrations are performed. This manipulation is excellent when the skin is very tender to touch, in addition to the painful underlying spasm.

Stroking and effleurage must be performed with great smoothness and no flourish of the hands at the beginning or end of each line of work. Kneading must be at sufficient depth not to tickle, and must be very even throughout the length of the line of work. Your hand movements between manipulations, must be calm and unhurried and within the tempo of the work being performed. It is sometimes advisable to tell the patient when a change of work is to be effected, but this should not be done when attempting to obtain general relaxation by treating either the whole neck and back, or by whole body stroking.

Whole body relaxation can sometimes be gained by performing a sedative massage to the back and neck, more especially so if the patient can be made comfortable in the prone lying position. Some patients find the use of an active technique of relaxation by some form of muscle action and relaxation, or by posture or by meditative methods impossible, and they may respond to whole body stroking. Ask the patient to remove some outer clothing, and to lie down either prone or in side lying. Cover him or her from neck to toes with a blanket, and tuck it in firmly over the neck. Take up a long, lunge standing position at the side of the plinth near the lower limbs (Fig. 1.1), and check that you can reach forwards to the shoulder and turn your hands and body to reach the feet (avoid the soles). Now work out a pattern, so that you stroke over every part of the body equally, e.g.

patient in prone lying—one hand each side of centre back
                                        —one hand each side over scapulae
                                        —one hand each side in line with axillae
                                        —one hand each side down arms and outer
                                            sides of legs

patient in lying—follow a similar pattern (use a curved line of work outwards or inwards round the breasts)

patient in side lying—either work single handed on the back or single handed on the front, or one hand each side covering opposite areas.

These patterns mean both hands work together, and you must exert good control over both your movements, posture and the downward pull you exert to keep the movement smooth and of even depth. The human body can have quite sharp hillocks and valleys when lying down for this treatment, and it is easy to do fast downhill runs and bump at the valley bottom.

Some patients prefer a single handed pattern of work—one stroke to the right and one to the left. This technique may be forced on a small practitioner treating a tall patient, when you will increase your reach by rotating your trunk as well as reaching with your upper limb.

A technique called 'thousand hands' is sometimes used to overcome reaching problems. Each hand in turn performs a short stroke, each stroke overlapping that previously performed by ⅔ of its length.

Total relaxation may be induced in some very tense patients by giving them a very slow facial massage, or by a sedative massage to the neck with the patient in lying as in Fig. 6.1. When using this position it is easily feasible to work on the suboccipital muscles, especially those forming the suboccipital triangle, and the position and technique is helpful for posterior tension headaches.

Massage in sport

Massage is a most useful adjunct in the preparation of any athlete for their sport, and a helpful follow-up after intense physical activity. It is especially useful when successive intensive activity is to be practised, as when athletes participate in a series of heats.

Pre-activity massage

The athlete should have a shower, initially warm, and then cooler before the massage. If a needle shower is used, then a period of rest of about half an hour should follow the massage. The needle shower should also start warm and finish cooler.

If the subject exhibits extreme tension, give a sedative back massage first, followed by massage to the muscle groups which will be used in the activity. For some sports all four limbs and the back may have to be massaged.

To induce relaxation, use long stroking down the back until you become aware of a change of tone in the muscles. Follow with increasingly deep effleurage and then with kneading. Finish with effleurage.

For the specific action area, start with deep effleurage at a moderate tempo, follow with kneading, picking up and muscle rolling and/or wringing as appropriate, then increase the tempo of your work repeating all the manipulations several times. Complete the work with some percussion, choosing appropriate manipulations for the part and with very brisk stroking down the whole length of the part.

In dealing with the lower limbs, it may be advisable to treat the posterior aspect with the patient in prone lying and work on the glutei, hamstrings and calf muscles, then ask the athlete to turn to the supine position and work on the quadriceps, adductors, anterior tibials, peronei and the foot.

For athletes who primarily use their arms and upper trunk, remember to treat the whole back, neck and shoulder girdle region as well as each upper limb.

The subject should experience a feeling of warmth in the part and be aware of a feeling of well being at the end of the treatment. He or she should rest for a period of time to allow the skin to cool down before starting training or competitive activity. Warm clothing should be put on before going out into cool outside air.

Post-activity massage

The athlete should precede the treatment with a warm shower and the activity muscles are then treated. The purpose now is to aid drainage and to aid removal of the high accumulation of waste products from the activity. The rate of work is much slower and initially, at a tolerable depth. If the muscles are painful, they must be handled with care to avoid further tension in them.

Start with slow, firm effleurage and increase the depth, but not the speed, as relaxation occurs. Follow with slow kneading, working on each muscle group in turn and with as much squeeze as is tolerable. As each muscle relaxes, increase the depth of work and gently roll the muscle from side to side, before further kneading and effleurage is given.

Avoid all percussive manipulations.

If there is local tightness or spasm, the athlete may exhibit signs of painful discomfort as you handle the area. He or she may exclaim, pull a face or go into more spasm. This indicates a need for a more gradual approach to the area. Work round it with short effleurage strokes, knead adjacent muscles and the non-painful parts of the muscle in spasm. Remember, a muscle consists of the contractile and non-contractile elements, and the latter may be treated by finger or thumb kneading, gradually encroaching on to the painful area. Sometimes, lateral rocking or rolling of the muscle is more tolerable than kneading, as these manipulations are less compressive. Keep interspersing your work with effleurage, until the muscle relaxes sufficiently to allow more squeezing manipulations to be performed, so that the waste products of activity can be squeezed out of the muscle. Finish with plenty of deep slow effleurage.

Painful spasm or cramp may also indicate damage such as occurs from accidental kicks or blows. If this symptom is exhibited in response to the trauma, gentle treatment as described above should be instituted, but be aware that such injuries can lead to haematoma, or tearing of the tendon, or even rupture of the muscle belly, in which case early massage is contra-indicated (see p. 104 on haematoma).

Bibliography

Beard, G. (1974) *Massage—Principles and Techniques.* Saunders, Philadelphia.

Creighton Hale, A. *The Art of Massage*, 2nd edn. Scientific Press, London.

Cyriax, J. (1941) *Massage, Manipulation and Local Anaesthesia.* Hamish Hamilton, London.

Cyriax, J. (1977) *Textbook of Orthopaedic Medicine*, Vol. 2, 9th edn. Baillière Tindall, London.

Ebner, M. (1985) *Connective Tissue Manipulations.* Robert E. Kreiger, Florida.

Gardner, E., Gray, D.J., O'Rahilly, R. (1969) *Anatomy*, 3rd edn. Saunders, Philadelphia.

Guthrie-Smith, O.F. (1943) *Re-habilitation, Re-education and Remedial Exercises.* Baillière Tindall, London.

Hollis, M. (1981) *Practical Exercise Therapy*, 2nd edn. Blackwell Scientific Publications, Oxford.

Hollis, M. (1985) *Safer Lifting for Patient Care*, 2nd edn. Blackwell Scientific Publications, Oxford.

Hollis, M. & Yung, P. (1985) *Patient Examination and Assessment for Therapists.* Blackwell Scientific Publications, Oxford.

Lewis, T. (1927) *The Blood Vessels of the Human Skin and their Responses.* Shaw, London.

Licht *et al.* (1963) *Massage, Manipulation and Traction*, 2nd print. E. Licht, Connecticut.

Mennell, J.B. (1940) *Physical Treatment by Movement, Manipulation and Massage*, 4th edn. Churchill, London.

Prosser, E.M. (1941) *Manual of Massage and Movements.* Faber & Faber, London.

Shires, I.C. & Wood, D. (1927) *Advanced Methods of Massage and Medical Gymnastics.* Scientific Press, London.

Tappan, F.M. (1961) *Massage Techniques.* Macmillan, New York.

Index